M000311341

Strength in My Storm

Faith & Breast Cancer

by
Michelle J. Perzan

Cover Design: Alicia White, Back of the Room Productions
Interior Design: MJ Schwader, Inspired Life Publications
Editor: MJ Schwader, Inspired Life Publications
Back Cover Photo: Shelly Porsch Chetty/SPCreative Photography

Dedication

This book is dedicated to my family who helped me find strength in my storm. I love you all so much and I am so thankful for each of you.

"But you are a chosen generation, a royal priesthood, a holy nation, a peculiar people; that ye should show forth the praises of him who hath called you out of darkness into his marvelous light."
1 Peter 2:9

Strength in My Storm

Acknowledgments

Aaron Perzan – The love of my life – I'm still so in awe of how God brought us together at a time neither one of us was looking or expecting to find our soul mate. I always prayed for someone, but when God put you in my life, it was beyond anything I had thought I wanted. Thank you for showing me how to be closer to God, how to be strong in my walk, and for seeing through my eyes into my soul and heart, despite my brokenness when you met me after losing my dad to cancer. You have been amazing through the past few years and I love how you love the boys and me. There's nothing I can say that can truly show you my heart and how thankful I am for you. I love you with all of my heart – you are "my lobster." Here's to fulfilling our prophecy as husband and wife as we go forward.

D3 - Daniel, David, and Dylan – You three boys are why I do what I do and why I will persevere through anything, because I will be there to watch you grow up, become men of God, and bless so many lives. I love each of you for different reasons; you are all so unique. I am thankful each day that you are my sons and super happy that God allowed me to be your mama.

Julie (Ju Ju Bean) Michieli – We've always had such a close sister bond; I believe it started when I was born on your 8th birthday – you wanted a bike, but you got me for a baby sister instead! You have shown me what strength is, courage, integrity, and love. You have always been there for me, for every problem I ever had, every struggle – and every victory. I have always looked up to you and admired you, and I am so grateful that you are my sister. I love you Ju Ju Bean. Thank you for all you've done for me; I'm so excited to give back to you now.

Danny Trakalo – Even though you are quiet and watch from afar, you have been there when I needed, in the most trying times. I'm thankful that you are my brother. I love you Dan Dan.

Max & Molly (MJ) Michieli – To my godson/nephew and niece, you have been the lights of my life since you were born. I have the most fun being Aunty Shell. You both have shown strength through adversity and I am so proud of you. You are on my family vision board and when I look at it, I work harder because I want to do for you like your mama has done for me.

AnnMarie Roberts – To my little "sister" who always has my back, always encourages me, and makes me feel like I can do anything. You are an inspiration to me with your amazing outlook, despite having your own struggles with MS. You truly are the example of having strength. I love your heart and your amazing kindness and I'm so thankful that you are a part of my family.

Precilla Calara – So grateful you met Aaron on the plane that day! Thank you for always seeing my potential and plugging me in so that I can be a better version of myself. Because of you, I became a part of the AWSC, which truly changed my life. I'm so thankful for you and Rey. God bless you both. Love you!

Lane Winsett and Debbie Sitton - Thank you for recognizing the drive in me, seeing my heart and my passion, and supporting me through all my struggles. I love you both.

Esther Spina – Thank you for seeing something in me that I didn't. You pushed me to get past my fears and you helped me become a better version of myself. You have believed in me since we met and you have been giving me a platform to speak at the Ambitious Women's Conference (AWC) and share my story of God's grace. For that I am so thankful. You are the epitome of an ambitious woman, full of integrity, passion, and genuine love for others. Thank you for taking calls from me and talking to me like a friend, helping me through my struggles. I truly respect and admire you and hold a special place in my heart for you. Biggest hugs – I love you.

Amy Applebaum – What an amazing coach you have been for me! Thank you for creating the AWSC with Esther; it has changed so many people's lives – especially mine. I believe God put it on your heart to choose me for the first spotlight call and I'm thankful that you did; that was the "TSN turning point" for me. I can't thank you enough for all the belief you have put in me, the "gentle" pushing me off of cliffs to get me out of my comfort zone and the "kick my butt" in gear sessions! Everything you give me is exactly what I need. You really have done more than help my business; you have changed me into a bold, courageous, ambitious woman who is afraid and does it anyway (just like you always say!). I love you and your amazing heart. Thank you for all you have done and for being a part of this journey – I look forward to what's next! Let's do this!!! ;)

Stephanie Watson – My sister from another mister! From the time we moved into the hood, you have been there for me. Our friendship has been easy and real and it's turned into you becoming family, along with all of your kids and your hubby. Thank you for always encouraging me, lifting me up, and wanting to see me succeed in all that I do. A true friend is someone who wants the best for you and pushes you to be bold and get it – and you have done that for me. I love you girl!

Johanna Beaver – Our two boys caused us to become friends, and I am so thankful for you. When I have needed someone to talk to or when it comes to raising our boys, you are always there. You are a strong, amazing, kind person with a beautiful heart. I'm thankful for all you do for our family. You and your kids are so special to us. You deserve the best and to be happy my friend.

AWSC Women – To all of you amazing ambitious women of the success club – there's no way to name each of you, but you are all so important to me. You have aided in my growth, pushed me and encouraged me to step out of my "box" and soar! You have prayed for me during my surgeries, cried with me during struggles, laughed with me, and celebrated with me over victories. This is one of the most amazing groups I have ever been a part of and I am blessed beyond words. Thank you, from the bottom of my heart.

BNI Katy – To my BNI group, thank you for becoming like family so quickly! I was shy coming there and you saw through that, accepted me, and have pushed me to grow and prosper. This group has been amazing for my business, my confidence, and for forming so many new friendships.

Cassandra Washington – For giving me the courage to become an author and walk forward on the path God has lit up for me. Thank you for taking me in on your book, *Emerge: Real Stories of Courage and Truth*, and teaching me how to strengthen my wings. You are a shining light to others and a blessing to me!

MJ Schwader – For encouraging me and showing me that people need to hear my story, then pushing me to go deeper to tell it. Thank you for your gentle process and for teaching me so much about writing. Working with you is such a pleasure and I'm excited to see what our next project will be!

Katy Toastmasters – Thank you for being so supportive through the past few years. You encouraged me to share my journey as I was going through it and you lifted me up every time.

Grayson Lakes Playgroup – Just wanted to let all of you mamas know how amazing you are! You welcomed me right away, and whenever I had appointments, surgeries, or trips, you all rallied together to help with the boys, food, or whatever Aaron and I needed. I have never met such an amazing group of neighbors who look out for each other and want to help with no strings attached. Super thankful for that first Fourth of July parade, where I discovered Bunco and created friendships with all of you! I love you ladies!!!

Crossings Community Church – You were there through our entire journey with breast cancer, and we couldn't be more thankful for all that you did as a church for us, through prayers, meals, and watching our boys during surgeries. May your church be blessed tenfold for all you did for our family.

Bonugli's – Sensei Jeff, Sarah, and Jan – I'm so thankful to have each one of you in my life. Thank you Jeff for seeing that inner "bumblebee" in me, and making me Den Mom at the dojo – that really meant the world to me. You taught me strength – mind, body, and spirit – so that when I was diagnosed, I was very well equipped. You and Grandmaster Cristobal Lopez have a very special place in my heart.

My mom and dad – Gemma and Elmer Trakalo – Even though neither of you are still on this earth, I want to thank you both for raising me to be an entrepreneur, as you both were. For always teaching me to be kind to others, to find the person sitting alone and make friends with them, and to see the good in every one and every thing. I wish you could see my family and how amazing my boys are. I know one day we will meet again, in Heaven. Until then, you are always in my heart and a part of me. Love, your baby, Michy.

Finally, I give all thanks and glory to God, the reason I'm writing this book. Thank you for giving me strength for each day and filling my storms with hope and joy.

"In all thy ways acknowledge Him and he shall direct thy paths." Proverbs 3:6

Strength in My Storm

Table of Contents

Preface

I am happy to share my story. A story that I never thought I would have the courage to endure, or to share. My story has enabled me to stand on a testimony of faith. And how can you have a testimony without a test? How can you have a message without a mess? Oh, yes, there was a mess. The last few years have brought a wave of emotions, challenges, adversities, victories, and yes, even failures; they all became lessons.

Having this opportunity to share my story with you humbles me. I hope that it gives you encouragement to know that you can stand in your faith, however that looks to you, and that you can be positive through whatever test that life is giving you. A major keystone for me was making a decision to be truly thankful each and every day.

I pray my story empowers you. It is my pleasure to serve you and I thank you for reading my story. May it bless you and guide you as you find strength in your storm, as I found strength in mine.

Strength in My Storm

Chapter 1
Getting the Call

Life can change in an instant. Two years ago, as I was sitting in
our rental house at my computer doing some paper work and
waiting for my three young boys – D3 (Daniel, David, and Dylan)
– to come home from school, I got "the call."

My family and I had moved two months before to Katy, Texas
for my husband Aaron's job. We were so excited because he was
finally going to be working onshore and we would see him every
night! This was amazing since the previous nine years he had
worked offshore and we saw him less than half the year. We had
been praying for a job change for years, and it all happened in
God's perfect timing. We were happily settling into our new life.

But in that one moment, my life was forever altered. One
second I was living a full life as a mother, wife, and entrepreneur.
The next, I answered the phone, and as I listened to the voice on
the other end, I knew nothing would ever be the same.

In shock, I hung up the phone, wondering how it is that it was
okay for me to hear the news on the phone, without checking if
there was someone – anyone – there to console me, to hold me, to
tell me I would be okay. Instead, they just gave me the news: "You
have breast cancer." I went numb.

Back home in Canada, I would have received the test results in
the safety of my doctor's office. But in the U.S., the expediency of
a phone call often overrules any emotional consideration. Looking
back on it, I realize now that I am thankful I got the results right
away. But that day, I wished I had someone there with me when I
heard those frightening words.

February 27, 2014 was the day I received the call. While my life
does not look the same, I can now say that I would never want to

go back. However, on that day, that outcome was impossible to imagine.

Devastatingly, at the same time, my mama was in hospice back in Canada, slowly and painfully dying of bone cancer. A few months before my life-changing phone call, she had back surgery to relieve the possibility of paralysis caused by tumors on her spine. She had not been doing well since then. I had just come back from seeing her, knowing it could be my last time with her, when I got my own news.

The tests that led to my own diagnosis were taken before I had left to see my mom. I am grateful that I did not know the news when I visited her. Seeing my mama in the shape she was in was heartbreaking, especially after seeing my Papa Smurf also suffer and die from cancer twelve years earlier.

All of my previous memories of loss surfaced as I was holding the phone to my ear. Receiving the call about my own cancer, all I could see was my dad, my mom, and my oldest brother Steven who passed away from Leukemia at the age of eight years old. I hung up the phone, trying to absorb what I had heard as the silence engulfed me… I had breast cancer. Now what?

Chapter 2
Coaching the Fear Out of Me

I am a work-at-home mom in a network marketing company where I help people save money and make money on electricity, and also with health and nutrition. Prior to the call, in November of 2013, I felt I needed to change how I worked in my business so that it would grow more.

One night I got a call from my business partner and friend Precilla, and she told me about a new Ambitious Women's Success Club (AWSC) that was launching. They needed a few founding members to trial it, and if I signed up by midnight, I could get in.

Having already been praying for God to open doors for me so I could grow my business, I knew this was an answer to those prayers. I hung up the phone and registered right away with my new coach, Amy Applebaum.

From there, I jumped in with both feet. Being introverted when it came to strangers, I knew I needed to be bolder and courageous, and I hoped Amy could help me. I could be fun and outgoing once I was comfortable, but to enter a room of strangers made me panic and get extremely nervous.

Amy did something called a Spotlight call with members once a quarter and we all had to send in applications showing why we wanted help and what we wanted help with. I sent in my application and I was picked to be the very first spotlight call on January 17, 2014.

I still remember finding out I was going to be the very first Spotlight call! I couldn't believe it and wondered how I was picked (to this day I still don't know how I was picked from so many – other than it was by the grace of God).

The call with Amy was a game changer for me. She had me dig deep, showing me that my fear of talking to people about my business was because I was so concerned about what they would think of me and how I would sound. I realize now that is a selfish point of view, but when I got nervous, I would stutter and then I would get self-conscious – then the sweating would start and soon I had no idea what the other person was saying! I was so busy thinking about something smart to say, and trying not to become a blabbering, stuttering mess, I wasn't really listening to them at all.

Amy showed me that I needed to truly connect with people first, with no agenda; that's how relationships are formed. After all, people like to do business with other people they know, like, and trust, right? For that to happen, I needed to start having genuine conversations, start asking questions, and be vulnerable – something I wasn't the best at. I liked holding everything inside way too much.

From a young child I held things inside, where it felt safe. There were times I didn't want to speak out because I thought I would be bothering people or that my opinion really didn't matter. Those were all negative thoughts and beliefs that I put on myself, and I played into.

Having Amy pull out my feelings in front of others, even though it was on the phone, made me nauseated and uncomfortable. I was better at smiling and putting on an act that everything was good, while staying in my "comfortable" corner watching everyone else.

When I finally let my guard down on the phone, I could feel walls breaking down because I was being honest and vulnerable. If I wanted to grow at all, I needed to do both. She kept prompting questions and asking me why I wanted to do this business, how it made me feel, why I wanted to help others. She showed me that I can't help anyone if I am not asking others questions, engaging in conversation, and really finding out how I might be able to help them.

Amy encouraged me to join Toastmasters (which has nothing to do with toast, I learned!!) and to engage in that and in talking with others. I was afraid to go to a place where I didn't know anyone, but I wanted to grow, so as Amy says, I faced fear and did it anyway. Best decision ever!

What a daunting feeling, walking in the first week of Toastmasters, not knowing anyone in a room of over 40 people. I just about passed out I was so nervous. I kept breathing and smiling, and then I made a goal to talk to one person and have a real conversation and learn about *them.*

Toastmasters is a place where different types of people from all walks of life come to become better speakers. From stay-at-home moms to CEO's, anyone who wants to be more effective at speaking comes to meetings. The group was diverse and amazing. I joined that first week, uncomfortable and all.

Just weeks after my Spotlight call, I received the call that I was diagnosed with breast cancer. There was an Ambitious Women's Conference (AWC) coming up at the end of March 2014, my birthday weekend, less than three weeks away, and I had just found out I had cancer. The AWC is a conference hosted by Esther Spina, one of our top women income earners, to provide women entrepreneurs a weekend of training.

Having been at this conference for the previous two years, I knew how inspiring and empowering it was, and each year I learned more about my business and me. If I wanted to grow personally and in my business, it was important that I was there.

Having just done the Spotlight call, and implementing the tasks Amy was giving me, I was growing personally. Amy and Esther asked me to give a brief testimonial at the up-coming AWC; sixty- to ninety-seconds about how the AWSC had been helping me. I said yes, even though that was *way* out of my comfort zone and made me want to throw up.

The weekend of the conference came and I was filled with fear. There were five of us on stage that were going to give our quick sixty-second testimonials. Just walking up to the stage, I started to sweat and feel nauseated, thinking how am I going to get through this?

Shaking, filled with shear terror on stage, Esther had to hold the microphone for me while I read off a piece of paper. That's how fearful I was of speaking in front of anyone. To share that I had breast cancer scared me even more; I was being vulnerable, something that was also very difficult for me.

The testimonial was for one-minute, but it felt like an eternity up there with over 500 women looking at me while I stammered through my part, just about in tears. I shared that my mama was in hospice dying and that I had been diagnosed with breast cancer three weeks before, but that having the support from the AWSC had been a blessing to me personally and to my business.

I am so thankful I was bold enough to share, because the entire weekend was filled with women praying for me, strangers becoming friends, and receiving hugs wherever I went. God showered me with love and showed His love and comfort for me being a yielded vessel, for sharing what I was going through, and for being vulnerable. I knew then that I had to be open about my entire journey, to let others in, and to be able to accept their help, love, and support by receiving it openly.

God puts the right people in your life at the perfect time – His perfect timing. Amy was not only put in my life to help me focus on my business. She helps me grow as a person, teaches me to be bold and courageous, shows me that I have a lot to give, and helps me be a better version of myself.

Amy is still my coach because she has not only helped in my personal development, but has shown me how to be an entrepreneur and a leader with integrity and honor, during the hardest time of my life. For that I will be forever thankful. I don't even know how the following weeks, months, or past two years would have been without her.

Chapter 3
I Will Praise You in This Storm

Four months before my diagnosis, I had my first mammogram in Harlingen, Texas, where we were living before we moved to Katy. The image had shown calcifications, and I had to go back to do a more intense mammogram, and an ultrasound, which led to a biopsy.

The results of the biopsy came back benign, but the surgeon told me to follow up with an oncologist to check my hormone levels when we moved to Katy. At the time, I thought it was a bit strange to follow up with an oncologist when I did not have cancer, but I didn't question it and that was what led me to self-refer to M.D. Anderson for them to check my hormone levels. Because I self-referred, they ended up re-doing all of my tests and taking more biopsies.

What was amazing was that the doctor who saw me said they didn't do hormone level checks and she was not sure why I was there. I still remember looking at her confused, and she had this genuine concern in her eyes. She went against protocol and reordered all of the tests so that they had a baseline, even though I had just had all the tests just four months before in Harlingen.

Because of her "gut feeling" and having the tests redone, I got the call back that I had cancer. Talk about God moving us to Katy in His perfect timing...

After getting the call that I had breast cancer, Aaron and I had to go back to M.D. Anderson and meet with everyone – the oncologist, radiologist, plastic surgeon, and surgeon. They went over so much information and options with us, it was overwhelming, to say the least. So much to absorb....

Aaron was amazing at taking notes, which was a good thing because the doctor would explain something and then go on to something else and I was still back at the first thing he had talked about!

Aaron would see my eyes glaze over as he kept taking notes, knowing I had no idea what was being said or what was going on. Taking it in all at one time, and with things in Canada as they were with my mama, I couldn't focus; it was too much. I kept waiting to get the call that my mom had passed away. That's not a way you want to live, but dreading the call was there in the back of my mind every day.

The doctors gave me a few choices. How do you choose between a lumpectomy, mastectomy, and a bi-lateral mastectomy? I didn't want to do any; I just wanted to go back to February 26th when I didn't know anything.

Sometimes they say ignorance is bliss, and it sure can be. However, this was not the time for that. Everything was happening so quickly, and I knew it was God opening doors and putting the right people in my path. I just was trying to breathe and get through it.

If you had asked me years before, I would have told you that I would *never* have surgery for anything; that it was not an option. I would have told you that anything and everything I would do would only be 100% natural. Remember that bible song, "Oh, be careful little mouth what you say"? As much as I didn't want to do any surgery, I knew that was not God's plan for me. I did not know the reasons, but He did.

For those few weeks while making my decision, I spent days and days walking around a pond by our house, listening to Christian music, and praying to God, asking Him to show me what to do. I listened a lot to *Praise You in This Storm* by Casting Crowns, and I would cry and shout out to the Lord asking for some sign.

Each morning I would drop the boys off at their school, come home, and walk and pray and cry and listen to music. I would cry out loud, and then I would be silent, as tears would stream down my face. Releasing the pain through crying felt good. I was mourning from not being able to speak to my mom in weeks, as she was too ill to talk on the phone, and I was trying to cope with the decisions that I knew God was showing me every day. I just didn't want to see or believe that it was true.

Every night I would have the same dream – the dream of a bi-lateral or "double" mastectomy. It was a peaceful and calm dream. It was God clearly showing me what my path was. Every morning I woke up and thought, 'that can't be right'. So, I would walk again the next day, cry, and shout out for Him to show me the right path. This happened for quite a while. I'm a tad bit stubborn, don't you think? I was praying for answers, God was showing me them, yet I was not open to receive what He was providing me.

Daily I would get into the shower, which was my safe haven, and cry my eyes out again in desperation. And then I would sing, "…and though my heart is torn… I will praise you in this storm…."

Strength in My Storm

Chapter 4
Am I Making the Right Decision?

After meeting with so many doctors, and seeing my family history, M.D. Anderson doctors had me in to have genetic testing within the week. I was and still am so amazed at how efficient and professional M.D. Anderson is when it comes to the beginning stages after finding out you have cancer.

After the testing, it takes up to four weeks to get the results. This not only affected me, but also my older sister Julie, who I call Ju Ju Bean, and my niece, who I often refer to as Little MJ (since I am Big MJ - Michelle Janis and she's Molly Julia); she holds a special place in my heart. If the results were positive, they would also need to go for testing, and, like me, have to make some very important life decisions.

Thinking I had all the answers, I thought if I had positive results I would just have all the surgeries, without another thought. That meant, the double mastectomy and hysterectomy. Which means, I wasn't going to rely on listening to what God wanted me to do. Not a shocker, since I wasn't listening anyway!

My thought was that I was already blessed with three healthy boys and I was done having children, so my health was most important. I planned to be around for my boys' graduation, their weddings, and their children. I would tell the doctors to take everything out!

Every day I proclaimed that I would be around to watch my D3 boys grow up. I believed that and I know it made a difference. The mind achieves what the mind believes. Isn't that what they say?

They had only found one small area with cancer – estrogen receptor positive carcinoma (ER 90%) – and that it was only stage

1, so as I mentioned, they said that I could either do a lumpectomy or a mastectomy, or a bi-lateral mastectomy, and gave me pros and cons for each. The decision was big for anyone to make, especially when still in shock from the diagnosis.

Before the results even came back and after much praying, I knew that a lumpectomy was not for me. I knew deep down in my gut – you know that feeling – that I had to have a bi-lateral mastectomy. It was only a week before the surgery that I came to terms with it after many, many walks around that pond, and many, many tears shed.

Looking back, I don't know why I was fighting the decision so hard. Part of me wanted control, upset that I couldn't make the decision myself. The other part of me couldn't imagine not having breasts anymore. How would I feel? How would I look? How would others look at me? What would Aaron think? I had worn a bra since grade five, so to just not even need one seemed so odd.

All my boys breastfed; how would it be not having them anymore? Would I still feel like a woman? I struggled so much with it because I thought maybe it would change me or how I would feel, or how others would look at me. That's how the world is, right? We judge each other by outward appearances before we even know the inside of someone.

So many thoughts went through my head, and even though in my gut I knew what the right decision was, my thoughts kept getting in the way of what God was showing me. My fear and control were in the way of seeing what God's plan was for me.

It's like God was preparing me for what was going to happen and what they were going to find. Each step of the way I had to trust in God, praying and praising Him through this storm, because I knew I wasn't alone. Each day I had to make a point of fighting off thoughts of "what if," and without prayer, I was not going to hear God's plans.

There were many prayer warriors lifting me up, and I'm so thankful that I had them and my husband on my side. I also had God, who would never leave me and would give me an abundance of strength to get through any trial, and to do it with a smile, since I was not strong enough to do it on my own.

Chapter 5
I Want My Mama!

When something bad happens, who do you automatically want to call? Your mama? Your dad? A sister, brother, or friend? There's usually someone you want to share news with, good or bad.

As I mentioned, my mama was suffering in hospice from bone cancer. She had been diagnosed almost four years before, the year my youngest son Dylan was born, and she fought like the stubborn Italian woman that she was. Another reason I admired her.

In early February 2014, I traveled back to Canada to visit my mom after my sister called me to let me know it might be the last time I could visit her while she was able to communicate with me. My heart spoke to me, and my gut said it was the right thing to do. I hopped on a plane, and was so thankful that I made the trip to see her.

That's one way I hear from God – that "feeling" in my gut that I know I need to do something. It's God nudging me in the right direction, and I'm so thankful for all my "nudges."

When I saw my mama, I knew that it was my last time with her. She had been in an induced coma, and by God's grace came out of it the night I arrived. I got to spend a couple of days with her and we were able to have a few moments of talking and prayer, which I loved.

With the medication affecting her moods, her memory, and her personality, even though I knew my mama was in there, it was not really her anymore. She was suffering from pain, and it was so hard for everyone to watch. I can't imagine what it was like for her. No one should ever suffer like that.

When people are put on medications, it can cause horrible side effects, which change or alter so many things. The person taking the meds feels out of control, and sometimes doesn't even remember what they said that was harsh, mean, hurtful, or rude. It's not them, it's the meds, but when you're around it for long periods of time, it's hard not to take it personally.

Watching my mom suffer and knowing in the back of my mind that I had tests taken to see if I had cancer weighed heavily on my heart. There was a part of me that wondered if that would soon be me lying in a hospital bed like her. Would I be suffering in pain? Would I be mean to others? Would I hurt loved ones without meaning to?

I was afraid to end up like her in hospice not knowing who was there to be with me while I moaned in pain – to lay helpless, not able to get up to walk, knowing it's the end of my life. I had to keep walking out of the hospital room to cry; I could hardly contain my fear sitting beside her watching her have hallucinations from the meds.

What a challenging week that was for me emotionally, especially once I left to come back home, knowing in my heart I would never see her alive again.

Once I got home and I was diagnosed with breast cancer, I called my brother Danny to let him know, and then I told my sister Julie. After talking with them, and considering how my mama was, we all thought it would be better if I didn't tell her. What would it help? It would only make her suffer more knowing her baby Michy had cancer (I am the youngest of 4 children), and there was nothing she could do. If I had known before I went there in February, I may have told her, because we would have been face-to-face. I really don't know. I just know that it wasn't right to tell her and make her suffer even more when I was so far away in Texas.

My heart longed to tell my mama, "I have breast cancer," and to hear her say, "It's okay Michy, you are going to be just fine." To have her tell me, "You're young and strong and you can beat this thing." That's what I wanted to hear. I knew with all the meds that she was on that she probably wouldn't have been able to say that, even if deep in her heart she felt it.

With all the rationalization in the world, there was that little girl in me that longed to tell my mommy and my Papa Smurf that I had cancer; to have her be the take-charge woman I know she used to be and have my dad give me his big bear hug and protect me and tell me what to do. As fantastic as it is to be able to talk to people about having cancer, there is really nothing like the comfort of a parent.

I know telling her would have been selfish, as much as I wanted her to be there for me like she had been so many other times. I knew that this time I had to lean on God and my husband and my other family and friends. But they still weren't my mom. That was such a hard thing for me.

In the meantime, I had reached out to prayer warriors all over, letting them know that I hadn't told my mama, but to pass on to anyone they knew who would pray for me. I have been very open about having cancer and allowing people to see that it does not have to define you or bring you down, that you can take control of your own life by proclaiming your own truth and taking the victory in Jesus Christ.

While being lonely for a parent, I was reminded that my Father in Heaven was right by my side, and He would comfort me through this storm. None of that comes easy; it's a daily commitment of praying, being positive, and persevering, even when your heart feels like it's breaking.

To this day, I still think that my mama knew "something" was wrong. I think it's mama instincts, or that "gut feeling" that you have with a child. The last few phone calls we had, she would ask me if there was something I wanted to tell her. All I would say is that I loved her very much and I missed her, and then I would ask if she wanted to pray. I would hang up and cry my eyes out, feeling like I was lying to her, yet knowing in this case, it was best for her. No one ever said that doing the right thing was easy...

Due to the meds, the calls slowed to a stop; her mind was just too muggy with the effects of the medication. She could no longer hold conversations and was hallucinating so much that she did not make sense. The doctors told me that bone cancer is one of the most painful of cancers, and to keep my mom comfortable they had to give her a lot of painkillers along with her other medications, so she was sedated most of the time.

So even though my mama was still alive in hospice, not being able to talk to her everyday like my boys and I were used to was a mourning process that started very early and caused me much anxiety, stress, and sadness.

Knowing someone is alive, but you can't talk to them or see them was just so difficult for me. Living so far away, knowing there was nothing I could do took a toll on me daily – I had to just keep praying for her and my brother and sister every day knowing that they were facing a huge storm themselves and having faith that they would find some peace of their own.

Chapter 6
Will Cancer Kill Me Too?

Watching my dad die from cancer and then watching my mom suffer, the emotional impact I was feeling was really more than I could describe. My heart still aches in pain from missing my dad so much – from what I wanted him to see in my life, what I wanted him to take part in – like walking me down the aisle, meeting my husband and my three boys, and seeing who I have become.

There are still days that I cry thinking of my Papa Smurf because I just want another day to tell him I love him. Then watching my mom become a different person as the meds took over her body and made her go from one of the most intelligent women I knew to a blabbering mess. Watching someone you love diminish in mind, body, and spirit takes such a toll on the family. And how could I not think – will I be next?

Knowing how I was grieving, I worried about my boys and husband. Would I experience what she was going through? Was I going to lay in a hospital bed and turn into someone who didn't remember anyone, not knowing what was going on, what day it was, or who was there?

Would I have to have someone wash me, dress me, or feed me? Would I be left alone in a hospital room night after night, with no nurses that really cared if I needed to be taken to the bathroom, or if I was hungry?

If I died, would my boys remember me when they grew up? Would they talk about me? Had I given them enough stories of my parents and family that they would remember? What legacy was I passing on to them? Would they miss me? Would they be okay; would I be okay?

Thinking of what it would feel like to be in that bed dying, to go through the pain my mom experienced freaked me out. I was scared, and I didn't want to leave my husband and my kids the way my parents had left me; they were too young and so was I. I wasn't ready to die. I begged God not to take me yet; I would do whatever I had to – whatever He said.

To think at 42 my life could end up like my parents and what a harsh effect that would have on my boys broke my heart. I had not done enough yet; it couldn't be the end for me. I had so much to learn, so much to still teach my boys, and so much to share with others.

Chapter 7
Walking with Faith

Even though I had the dreams to have the bi-lateral mastectomy, does not mean it was an easy decision to make. Being shown something by God and actually listening and doing it are very different.

There was so much that I was still holding in, even though I felt I was being much more vulnerable. I was having a challenge giving up control of what would happen and it was causing me inner turmoil that I didn't really talk about with anyone.

Questions would pop in my head, and fear and my inner issues of trust would come into play. I was afraid of what would happen during surgery. What if I didn't make it? What if my boys were without a mama? What if afterward Aaron did not desire me or love me anymore? If I died, would my boys remember me? Would Aaron re-marry? Would *she* be their new mom? Did I do enough for my boys?

If you were just diagnosed with breast cancer, what would go through your mind? How would you feel? To be honest, you can't even answer that until it really happens to you. Before I was diagnosed, I had my own thoughts of what I would do; but none of that happened in reality. Those thoughts in my head – fear, total and complete fear – were lies from the enemy that were creeping into my mind. I was doing all I could to hold that enemy off, but my mind was racing too fast and furious to control it. Oh, yeah, control, that issue just kept popping up!

Control issues for me came from when I was a child. An adult touched me indecently when I was around six years old. He was a work colleague of my dad's and he came to town every so often and would stay with us instead of in a hotel. Being the snuggly, affectionate person that I was, I wanted to sleep with him, not thinking anything of it, as I was a young child.

One night, he touched me indecently and when I reached out for help, initially no one believed me. My sister was the one who took me to my mom and made me tell her. But back then, you didn't talk openly about it like you do now.

I believe because it was a business friend, nothing was ever said. My dad was never told until I was in my 20s, so I felt like my voice did not matter. So my trust, control, and fear issues arose early in my life. I felt I had a lack of confidence from being violated and then having my experience dismissed at such a young age.

Then when I was 14, my "boyfriend" at the time raped me. I believe that it was my lack of confidence and respect for myself that led to this happening, even though I know it was not my fault. After it happened, he called and left a message on my answering machine, breaking up with me. I cried for days.

I never told a soul about the rape until I was 33, when I shared it with my husband. After what happened when I was a child, I didn't think it would matter and I really thought it wasn't rape, because he was my boyfriend. Only later did I learn that no means no, whether it's a boyfriend or stranger. It was not my perfect idea of my "first time," but it was definitely something that I would never forget.

I eventually spent time with a psychiatrist, I went to a hypnotherapist, and finally in my 20s I was able to face my demon – the one who hurt me when I was a child – and confront him.

In that moment I was a terrified little girl again, but I had to face him and ask why. But there was no point, since he said something along the lines of, "...it's not like I had sex with you." As if that made it somehow better.

These two parts of my life caused a control issue with me. In those two situations I had no control over what was happening to me. So I felt from that time on I needed to control everything I could and feel some sort of safety.

I was able to forgive both of them and moved on... or at least I thought I had moved on. Until I got my diagnosis, and the fear rolled back in and the scared and vulnerable girl came back.

If I were in surgery, where would my boys be? Who would get them to school? Who would tuck them in? Would they pray with them? Would they snuggle them the way they like? What would they discuss with the boys? I was so busy trying to control how everything would go that I stopped trusting in God, which would have taken my fear away.

We had just started going to a new church, so we barely knew people there. We attended a small group and liked the couples. I knew these were probably some of the people that would take care of my boys, but who else would be there for them? Where did they live? Would it be safe? What shows would they allow them to watch? How about showers? Would they brush their teeth, and would they eat any of the foods they liked? Would they have enough to eat? The thoughts at first were almost comical. I was living and thinking in fear instead of trusting in God.

Could I trust in God and still have fear? I don't believe you can do both. When you are constantly worried and fearing the outcome of something, how are you placing your trust in God? You aren't.

How could I worry about my boys being okay and where they would be when I was saying with my mouth that I trusted in God? That's not trust, that's fear, and when I was blinded by that fear how could I see God bless me and allow Him to show me *His* greatness?

We all have fear about things every day; that's normal and it happens. However, how we treat that fear is how we show our faith. When we acknowledge the fear, and see it, we can lean on God, ask for His guidance and strength to get through whatever is causing the fear, and then we can walk forward. When you see the fear that is crippling you or holding you back and you face it, you can overcome it because you stood up to it. When you do that, it will no longer have the same kind of power over you it once did.

When I get into my van to drive, I don't fear an accident, or something bad happening when I pull out of my driveway; yet it's a possibility every time I drive. Instead I stand in my faith knowing God's hand of protection is around me and I trust in Him to guide me.

The opposite of love is fear. And God cannot live where fear dwells. Truly, any negative emotion can be brought back to fear. Are you sad? That's fear of loss or losing someone. Are you angry? That's the fear of being like that person or being hurt. Those low-frequency emotions always lead back to fear. But fear *is false evidence appearing real* – it's natural to be fearful, and we all fall into the trap of believing that the fear is greater than the outcome! I know I sure did!

This had to be dealt with, so again, I prayed and asked God to give me His strength, to give me clarity on what to do, for me to completely trust Him, and for me to be able to feel His love and comfort. It was consuming me on the inside. I knew I couldn't properly heal if I was still holding things inside and pretending that I was okay.

The next day in church I went up for prayer to have peace about choosing the bi-lateral mastectomy surgery – to truly accept it. By the end of the day, I really did have peace. I knew God's hand was on me; I could feel it. I could feel everyone's prayers. I could feel the calmness come over me, and I knew it was the right decision. I was finally letting go of my issues of control and trusting in the Lord.

To go from that amount of fear and lack of trust to feeling peace is only by God's amazing grace – there was no other explanation of it. It was one of the few times that I just let go of everything my mind was thinking. It was such a challenge for me to do, but when I did, the freedom it gave me was empowering – it was like a dam broke, and I felt such joy.

The next morning, I called M.D. Anderson to tell them I decided to go with a bi-lateral mastectomy, and they told me that they already had me down for that. Isn't that interesting. God had it all worked out and all I could do is praise Him in this storm and thank Him once again for His love and for being all-powerful.

Chapter 8
Surgery

Going to my pre-op appointment for the breast cancer bilateral mastectomy on April 14th, 2014, I had no idea what to expect. I thought I would have blood work, talk to some people, and be done, then go home, even though they went over it with me beforehand that it would be much more involved than that. It's amazing how much information you forget when you are going through a difficult situation.

After blood work, EKG, and all the other tests, they sent me for a lymphoscintigraphy (yeah, I can't say it either). The procedure would include putting a needle in the left breast where they found the tumor and injecting liquid, and then an hour later, check the machine (MRI I think – again, it's all a blur) to be sure they could see the "liquid" draining into the lymph nodes. They do this so that the next day during surgery they can see where the "liquid" drained to and then check the lymph node to see if the cancer had spread.

Being there for pre-op, I was still in a daze, knowing that the next day my life would change in so many ways. I would be different, inside and out, good and bad. I also had a strange calmness over me, knowing that I was in the exact right place and I had the right doctors. I can honestly say it was a time where I actually felt God's perfect peace over me, even though my head was scattered, thinking a mile a minute.

At one point I told Aaron where I had put the will. Aaron would not even listen to me; he reminded me of our blessing from our marriage and that it had not been fulfilled yet, that God had lots left to do with both of us. When we were married, his Uncle Mario, who was a pastor, prophesied over our marriage and us at the church. He prayed in tongues and then brought forth a message from God. Among other things, he spoke of how we would go forward together and minister to many. We hadn't done that yet – not even close. So, I pushed all that negativity to the side, trusted my husband and God, knowing that everything would be okay. Visualizing positivity, I prayed that I would wake up to find that my surgery would go better than even the doctors could imagine.

Getting ready for any surgery can be difficult. But when we have someone with us who is encouraging and reminds us of what we should be focusing on, it can make all the difference in the world. I'm so thankful that Aaron was such a rock during all the appointments and procedures. He kept everything light-hearted and fun. It was *exactly* what I needed in my storm.

April 15th, 2014, I went in for my bi-lateral mastectomy, with Aaron by my side and people from church taking care of our three boys. Before we left for the hospital, the cutest pregnant lady, Kimberly, came to watch our boys. I did not meet her until that moment.

Oddly enough, my spirit was calm, a perfect peace you can only experience when you put all of your trust and faith in God. Knowing that my boys were "somewhere" with "someone" for the next 24 hours did not even phase me in that moment; I just knew that God had it covered and I truly trusted in Him.

The operating room was a blur – I remember being wheeled in on the bed, and them asking me to sit up so they could give me a block to help with the pain. Then I think I told a joke (go figure!!!), and then it was good night Irene!

Waking up I remember seeing Jackie, one of the nurses for the plastic surgeon. Later she told me I had given her thumbs up and a smile! During the surgery they removed all of the tissues from the breast and the nipple, and they also put in expanders, which would aid in my reconstruction process.

The surgery had two different surgeons; one doing the bi-lateral mastectomy and then the plastic surgeon came in to put in the expanders. The expanders are taken out months later and saline implants would be put in to complete the reconstruction.

After surgery, I was all smiles – because of the block and drugs, I'm sure! They brought me to recovery to be greeted by Aaron and my friend Rosie. What beautiful faces to see! I really don't remember too much about what I was saying, but many people helped me with those memories later.

Upon waking I asked two important questions, because they still stand out. One – was my mama still alive, and two, did they have to take out the lymph nodes? Aaron had a strange look on his face. He was like – that's what you're going to ask first thing? I could already tell by looking in his eyes that something was wrong, I just didn't know which question it related to.

My husband, knowing that if I ask the question, that I want to know the truth, told me what happened during surgery. The good news, my mama was still alive.... That meant the other news was there was more cancer....

When they went in, they had checked the one lymph node and it tested positive for cancer, so they took out 31 lymph nodes on my left side. When they were doing the bi-lateral mastectomy they found another tumor in my left breast that hadn't shown up in earlier tests. It was a more aggressive tumor, metastatic cancer. Now, instead of one cancer, carcinoma, there was the sneaky metastatic form, and there was the lymph vascular invasion. That was like speaking a foreign language to me. All I knew is that I wasn't fighting just one.

When Aaron was telling me this, I remember thinking how happy I was that I listened to that "gut feeling" I had – "God's voice" – telling me that the lumpectomy was not enough and that I needed to do the bi-lateral mastectomy.

Part of me was in shock realizing that there was more cancer in my body and the doctors didn't know and the tests hadn't shown it. There was a moment of panic where I thought, how did they not see more cancer with all the tests and the technology?

I could feel my body tense up and my mind racing as my thoughts and anxiousness were coming over me. But the greatest feeling I had in that moment was that of thankfulness. What if I hadn't done the bi-lateral mastectomy? What if I hadn't listened to what God was showing me? I would've had to have another surgery once they found that spot, weeks or even months later, and then what would my cancer have been – a stage 3 or 4?

Soaking in the news was overwhelming at first and then I stopped, calmed my thoughts, and focused on what I did correctly. I was thankful that they found all the cancer, I was thankful that they took out everything, and I was thankful that I was obedient and "listened" to what God was showing me to do. I was thankful deep in my soul...

The last thing I ever wanted to do was have a bi-lateral mastectomy – I mean what woman would want to? I also could not imagine if I had gone with a lumpectomy and in a few months or more found out I had another tumor all along, and have to go through another surgery.

If I would have gone by what I wanted, or what was suggested by the doctors, and worried about how I did not want to suffer, or lose my breasts, or look sick or different, things would have been so much worse. That was a humbling moment for me that showed that I am not in control of anything.

Often we make decisions based on fleshly things and shallow things and in the light of eternity does any of that really matter? Who cares if I have no breasts? Who cares if I would have had to do chemo and lost my hair? Who cares what strangers think when they look at me? Let's be honest, there's a part of all of us that cares; it's human nature, it's how we are.

But when I look at my husband and my boys and I see them, they are what matter to me. If I have no hair, but I'm with them, then I'm still a blessed and happy woman. If I have no breasts, but I still get to make love to my husband every night, then why should I care? It's all perspective and what really matters is in your heart.

Chapter 9
Coming Home

Recovery is always more painful than you think it will be. In the hospital they were giving me morphine for the pain, which upset my tummy. I could not keep any food down, not even liquids! So, my one night stay in the hospital turned into two nights. But it's like God was giving me extra rest for what was about to happen.

Aaron stayed the first night with me in the hospital, but the second night I told him to go and get some rest, since all I did was sleep and throw up. For the first time in forever I did not turn on the television for two straight days. I kept apologizing to the nurses for getting sick because every time they sat me up or brought me Jell-O, my tummy said NO!

The coolest thing about the hospital – they had a menu that you could order whatever you wanted! *A menu!!* That was totally stellar! The only unfortunate thing was that I couldn't order any food from it because I couldn't keep anything down! I remember being in the hospital in Canada after giving birth to my first son Daniel and there was no menu, so I loved the option of being able to order food, even though I couldn't eat. See, there's always a positive way to look at things.

On April 17th, Aaron got to bring me home, which was also his 33rd birthday, so he was excited for that present! I had already ordered his present online, knowing surgery was coming up. I was hoping it would be delivered by the time we got home from M.D. Anderson. He loves those old black and white wing tipped shoes, so I bought him a pair and knew he would just flip out when he saw them.

Aaron brought me home, then brought the reclining/rocking chair into the bedroom, along with a table and some nice cold water with ice and set me up all comfy with the remote. As soon as I sat in the chair, Aaron's cell phone rang. I knew it was "the call."

On the way home, we had called my sister Julie and told her we were on our way home and that I was doing good and that I had finally kept down some food. I told her once I got home, I would call her and let her know I was settled in. Well... she called first.

Aaron looked at me, and I knew my mama had passed away. It was just before 1 pm and I sat there stunned.

I thought to myself that it was like my mama knew. Even though I never told her about my cancer or my surgery, it's like she was a mama until the end. She waited until my surgery was over and until I was home safe and settled, before she found peace and rest at last.

The next day was Good Friday. Yep, it was Easter weekend, so they were not able to talk to anyone to set up anything for the funeral until Monday. I had my follow-up appointment on Monday with the surgeon, so I knew I would have to sit tight over the weekend, rest and recover, and then go Monday and ask for clearance to travel to Canada for the funeral.

Pain filled my body from the surgery I just had, but now the pain moved to my heart, where it broke a little more with the loss of my final parent. Even though I had been waiting for the call and I had not talked to her in weeks, it was so final; I could not believe she was gone. The woman who was stronger than anyone I have ever met (other than my sister Ju Ju Bean) and was just like Marie Barone (from *Everybody Loves Raymond*) was actually gone and I would never talk to her again. Tears streamed down my face, yet I did not make a sound.... It was the sign of a broken heart.

Again, only by God's grace would this happen on this exact day. Because it fell on a holiday weekend and they could not make any arrangements, it gave me that many extra days to recover. God knew my heart and that I wanted and needed to be at her funeral. Again, as heartbroken as I was, I had to smile with a thankful heart, because I knew that was God's doing. He was making a way for me to be able to travel to Canada to be at the funeral. I was getting three extra days of healing so that I would be able to travel, so how could I not be thankful even though this was a big storm.

Aaron and I decided not to tell the boys about Nona passing away that day. I wanted their daddy's birthday to be about him and happiness, because he is the love of my life. We had a small celebration, considering I just got out of the hospital. We waited a couple of days and then we told them Nona had passed away. That was not an easy conversation.

Strength in My Storm

Chapter 10
Safe Travels – Alone

Going to the doctor on Monday morning after Easter Sunday for my first follow-up after surgery made me a bit anxious; all I wanted was clearance to travel. Right away, I informed them that my mama had passed away, that the funeral would be that week, and would it be okay if I flew? They had told me after the surgery that I could not lift anything or raise my hands above my head. With that information in mind, they said I was healing amazingly well, and gave me clearance to travel!

The doctor and nurse were actually able to take out two of the five drainage tubes, and replaced the humongous tubes for some nice, small travel tubes, which would make life a bit easier for me. They also recommended getting "wheelchair" or medical needs on my ticket, since I just went through a surgery and that way I could get wheeled to the gates. Thank goodness for that, since I had no idea how out of shape I would be from the surgery! Not only that, I was not in the mindset to be walking and have people bump into me with how sore I was from the waist up.

Aaron had booked my flight for April 23, the prayers were April 24, the funeral was April 25, and I would come home April 27 for another appointment April 30th with the surgeons. I knew I could do it, even though part of me did not want to fly alone or be alone at such a hard time. But I knew that God would be with me every step of the way, giving me the strength I needed.

My cousin Teresa, who lives in St. Louis, was going up for the funeral, so we decided to meet in Chicago and then fly the last leg together; that way I wasn't alone and she could help me. Taking the painkillers caused me to forget everything, including my name, so I couldn't take them. I took a big bottle of extra strength Tylenol with me, taking a mega-dose every four hours. I was still in pain, but nothing was going to stop me from going to say my final good-bye to my mama.

Let's just say that things didn't work out the way they were supposed to. Teresa was on standby and could not get to Chicago, so I ended up traveling alone. I never told my sister she didn't make it because my sister was flipping out that I was even traveling after surgery, never mind alone. My sister would check in with me and ask if I was with my cousin and I just said, "Of course." I did not want her to panic or worry, because I was okay. I was at the gate, in a wheelchair or in the wheelchair area with people all around to help me if I needed it.

It's funny how Julie and Danny (my sister and brother) both did not want me to come. They didn't want me to travel after surgery. They were worried about infections and that I had drainage tubes in, and just felt I should stay home. For me, while I was going through all of this, it would be so hard for me to hear that someone was "worried" about me. When they said that, I wondered why? Is there something I am missing and don't know? It would make my mind turn to where it should not go.

This taught me the importance of words and sensitivities and how they can affect others. It's so important to me when someone is hurting or facing a storm, to encourage them, lift them up, and pray for them. When we give it to God, there is no need to worry!

My sister and brother made it very clear that no one would be offended if I didn't come and that they completely understood. That made my heart feel amazing; it was very kind of them after everything they had to go through with my mom during the past few months. They were the ones who were with my mama every day in hospice, putting up with the med's effects, and bearing the burden that took a toll on both of them. For them to be so kind to me after I had already missed doing "my part" with my mama, really showed me how amazing my siblings' hearts are.

At no time did I ever think I wouldn't go to the funeral. When I prayed, I always asked God to see my heart, and that if He could, to make it possible for me to go and be at the funeral. I needed to see everyone and say good-bye. I needed the closure.

Being so far away, it's like you're not part of what is going on, like it's not real. Being at the funeral would make it real for me. It made me really see that she was gone. Being at her apartment for the last time, looking at her things – her dishes, her cups, her pictures – things I just wouldn't really see again in the same way. I just felt in my soul that I needed to be there.

Standing in my faith, I knew I could get through the flights and the travel alone. I had God with me at all times and He already provided a way for me to go and say my good-bye to my mama. I just had one small thing to deal with before I left – looking at myself in the mirror.

Emotionally, surgery is the easy part; it's post-surgery they don't prepare you for. No one tells you about how you will look after the surgery and how your body will feel completely different. No one explains that your life will never be the same with showering, dressing, or sleeping because your body is drastically changed.

Once you're diagnosed with breast cancer, you focus on how to get better, and the daily positive outlook to be able to keep it all together. You don't think about what it will be like after surgery, once they've taken your chest, cut it open, and left nothing but scars to see in the mirror.

Once I got home I had no idea how I would shower with drainage tubes hanging from my body. It was hard enough sleeping, and now I had to figure out a way to get myself in the shower. It seemed like the most daunting task.

Then, in the most perfect timing, I received an amazing gift in the mail from a breast cancer survivor named Julie. She made it for wearing around your neck while you shower, with "clasps" on it to hook all of your drainage tubes to.

While you were dressed, your drainage tubes would be safety pinned on your clothes, hospital gown, whatever it was you were wearing; but showering while holding the tubes is quite a challenge. This gift was a blessing. These are the small things that they don't tell you about or prepare you for, yet it's a reality you need to face every day.

The day before I left for Canada, I had a huge breakdown in the bathroom with Aaron. It was right after a shower. He was drying me off and he was showing me what to do with the bandages and tubes so I could teach my sister how to do it while I was there.

Yes, that's right, my husband was my nurse through all of this. He was gentle and methodical and the best caretaker I could have asked for – something that I bet many spouses wouldn't even consider doing, and he did it with love and kindness. That is something I will be forever grateful for.

That day, April 22, was the first day I even looked at my scars and what was left of my breasts. It was the first time I put my hands on them and touched the skin, and I cried as I saw myself in the mirror. It was the first time I was acknowledging how I looked. It had been exactly seven days, and it was about time.

Looking in the mirror I didn't even recognize who or what I saw. My chest was completely flat, with horizontal scars across my chest where my breasts used to be. It was shocking and ugly and it scared me. I couldn't even look at myself; it was like a terrible accident and I didn't want to look directly at it.

Touching the skin was surreal. I could see I was touching it, but it was numb to the touch, so it seemed as though I was touching someone else. A feeling of horror and sadness washed over me as I looked at a body I did not recognize, in disbelief over what was in front of me. I felt I looked terrible, like a 10-year-old, flat-chested girl, who had been horribly cut up. I could not stop the tears.

Aaron stood beside me and told me how beautiful I was and how well I was healing. I couldn't believe how comforting he was, looking at me the way I was. It was his daily love, affection, and encouragement that got me through each day.

His "chasing me" like a schoolboy because of his desire for me brought my confidence back sooner than expected. One of the most helpful things for me was to start having sex as soon as possible and as much as possible, daily was best. Even though our chests could not touch and it was different at first, this made me see that I was still a woman, still desirable, and still wanted – so important after losing your breasts, especially the way I felt when I looked at myself – when I could look at myself.

That was one of my hardest days, having to face what happened, what I lost, physically and emotionally, and really turn to my faith for strength. It needed to happen so that I could face my next challenge – traveling to my mama's funeral. Crying can be so healing and cleansing, like the rain – and I *love* the rain.

Like the quote says, "Life isn't about waiting for the storm to pass. It's about learning to dance in the rain."

Living life really is about cherishing each day, finding good in each moment, and truly enjoying what you have. It's really the little things that make a difference – the prayers, the love, encouragement, and friendships… and contraptions so you can shower! Yep, true story!

Strength in My Storm

Chapter 11
Be The Beacon of Light

Being at the prayers in Canada for my mom was emotionally very hard. She was born in Italy, and came to Canada when she was eight. We have a huge family in Canada, and I knew I would get to see relatives I had not seen since my wedding almost ten years before, some even longer.

Flying in the night before the prayers, I got to my sister's house and Julie had bought butterfly necklaces for my niece MJ, for herself, and for me. My mom adored butterflies and the necklaces were tokens that my sister thought would be special if the three of us wore them. It was special and I loved the thought. The symbol signified a special bonding moment for the three of us that no one else would even see. There have been a few days since then that I have worn that necklace, when I feel I need extra strength or just to honor my mama, and it makes me feel close to her, my sister, and my niece.

My sister also gave me a special ring that my mom wanted me to have – a ring my dad gave her on her forty-second birthday. The last few times I spoke to my mom on the phone, while she was still coherent to speak, she kept telling me she couldn't wait to see my face when she gave it to me. She never did get to see my face, but the memory of the ring, which to me represents my mom *and* dad, is beautiful.

The irony is that my dad gave my mom the ring on her 42nd birthday and at the age of 42 I received it, after finding out I had breast cancer and losing my mom.

At the funeral home, I didn't even want to look at my mom. It had been a week since she passed away and she just didn't look like her. To be honest, I just didn't want to face it or accept what was happening that day. I traveled all the way there to be in denial of where I was and what I was doing.

Trying to stay strong, I sat in the front pew with my brother and sister and their spouses. And then the people came; a couple hundred were there, each giving their love and sympathies and kind words. There I was, with tubes hanging from me, hoping no one grabbed me too hard, as my chest (or what was left of it) was very, very tender and sore.

Instead of focusing on what was happening, I wanted to enjoy seeing everyone I hadn't in so long. Before I even entered the prayers, I prayed for God to give me strength and to not make it about me, but to give comfort to others. Knowing God provided a way for me to be there, I had to be a beacon of light and share what God had provided, and praise Him through it all.

For Italians, when someone passes away, they have "prayers" the night before, where everyone comes to view the body and pray and give condolences to the family. Usually the priest is there and he also has a short mass with songs. All the family was in the front pews, so I stood up for many of the older relatives and smiled at them and told them how nice it was to see them, thanking them for coming – and I meant it from my heart. As people went up the middle aisle, viewing my mom, and then came to hug us, Andrea Bocelli was playing in the background, and I couldn't help but smile; my mama loved him, as do I.

My heart loved seeing everyone, and remembering the old days and times with my mom and dad with each of these people that came. I loved to hear stories and see the people whose lives she touched. Having the mindset of being thankful for seeing everyone and making it about that instead of being sad about something I could not change made the night easier.

The other amazing thing about Italian families is that they can get the word out quick, and they are sure to pray for you. Once my mom passed away, my sister let a few family members know what was going on with me, to give a heads up in case I didn't travel for the funeral. All you have to do with good Italian families is let the head of each family know, and everyone will know ASAP! True story!

This was great, because almost everyone at the funeral knew I just had breast cancer surgery, and they were gentle with me. They asked how I was recovering, and seeing that I looked good gave them comfort.

When they asked how I was coping, I kept giving all the credit and glory to God. That to me is the best example of God and His glory, when so many people could see that I just had a bi-lateral mastectomy the week before, yet I was there. I had a smile and I was able to travel alone because God provided and gave me strength.

Picture this, it's April 25th, 2014, you wake up in the morning, knowing you have to go to your mama's funeral that day and you look out and all you see is white! It had snowed!

I had slept on the couch that night, the most comfortable for me, since after the surgery I could only lay on my back. Then I turned to see my sister in the kitchen – with no power. All the power was out on all of her street. Just writing this, I'm still laughing thinking about it!

We were shocked at first, and then I thought, 'Yep, of course! Mama wanted to make sure everyone remembered the day of her funeral, so she had to go out with a huge snowstorm and a big bang!' At least that gave us all something to smile about and laugh a bit, which our family seems to do in hard situations.

I believe that if you don't have a sense of humor about things, you will have a very hard life. You have to be able to laugh at yourself and situations, and find something good and something funny in all of it, or life is just too darn hard.

We found out that there was power at the funeral home and church, so we got up, my nephew Max drove to get coffee and tea for everyone, we fixed ourselves up the best we could without hot water, and waited for the limos to come and get us and take us to the funeral home.

Good thing my Aunty Adele and Uncle Walter were up from Rossburn, Manitoba for the funeral with their motor home so that we could use their plug-ins to fix our hair a bit!

We went to the funeral home, where we would say our last goodbyes. The pallbearers were there as well; all of my mom's nephews. I really still didn't want to deal with it or see her – it was like I was stalling the inevitable.

So off we went in the limos through the snow-filled streets to the church. We stood in the lobby as we waited for the pallbearers to bring in her coffin. I was fine until the coffin went in front of me and I looked in the church to see every pew filled with the faces of family, friends, and loved ones. I broke down in tears and could not stop crying. I couldn't even look up because I just could not see anyone's face. My brother Danny grabbed my hand and held it tight, which is exactly what I needed in that moment.

All the way up the aisle to the front pew I looked down, trying to stop myself from crying. I just couldn't believe where I was and what was happening. I kept wondering why I couldn't have cried last night or this morning in private!

That was the point where it just all seemed like it was too much: surgery, traveling alone, power outage, funeral – too many things at once. My heart and mind were exhausted and I felt like I was going to lose it.

Crying in that way was one of the first times I let my emotions go, where I was raw and vulnerable for everyone to see. I needed to do it, a wall I needed to break to continue with my healing.

Having my brother hold my hand through it all really helped. Then I had to stop and remember Aaron telling me that it's okay to cry and to just be me. He told me he wanted me to go there and be a shining beacon of light to others. It's amazing what he sees in my heart and in me.

Needless to say, I did get through it, because I was not alone; I never am because I always have God and my family with me.

After the service, my mom's grandchildren and godchildren gathered in the blowing, cold snow to say a final good-bye. She had wanted them to put carnations, her favorite flower, on her coffin. We shook our heads as we smiled and thought to ourselves, 'Yes, Mama Gemma, we won't forget this day.'

That's why I keep praising God in this storm, because He is fair, He is loving, He is always with me and He gives me strength to get through anything. To this day, I still look back and can't believe all of that really happened; it almost seems like a sad dream.

Chapter 12
Traveling After Surgery

Looking back, when I think about how I traveled to Canada after my breast cancer surgery, I wonder how I did it. When you are young and "look" healthy, it's interesting how people look at you when you are in a wheelchair or in a section that is for disabled people only. It's a great lesson about not judging people based on how they look.

When I was traveling, I had on my husband's shirt so it was hanging down pretty long; you could not see the drainage tubes dangling, as I had them pinned to the inside. I was walking *slowly* whenever I got out of the wheelchair, and I'm sure that it was odd to see.

When I got to the gate and sat at the "handicap" chair, the number of people who stared and then started whispering and giving me dirty looks was amazing. When I say whispering, I could clearly hear them, along with others sitting within earshot. I guess they wanted to be discreet, while still making sure I heard that what I was doing was disrespectful.

They were saying that they couldn't believe I would take the seat away from someone who actually needed it. How I was being selfish wanting to be up close so I could be in line first, and that I was very rude. That they couldn't believe a young girl, traveling alone would need to be hogging the handicap area, and that I probably just wanted to get in front to grab a window seat.

Hurt, I just kept my head down and sat there, knowing that they didn't know better, and that I couldn't take it personally. I wanted to turn around and explain that I just had a bi-lateral mastectomy and was traveling to my mom's funeral in Canada, but

I was honestly in so much pain and in such shock, that I just sat there, and instead prayed… a *lot*.

Even walking to the bathroom, someone would smile at me and then they would notice the tubes hanging out; it was amazing how quickly they looked away and got away from me. I felt like someone with a real handicap must feel daily – being treated differently because of how you look or something you have on – even when it's not your choice. That was so difficult.

On one flight when they called people that needed extra help to come up first and I got up, they all kind of stopped and watched me. Oddly enough, even the airline worker took a double look at my ticket and then looked me up and down. I just smiled and thanked them. What else can you do?

On the way home in the Toronto airport, they wheeled me from the plane, through customs, and to the security area. At that point I would walk through and then they would have a wheelchair for me at the other side to bring me to my gate.

They instructed me to sit in the "handicap" area and that someone would be there shortly for me. So, I sat and waited. Many workers walked by me and no one stopped. Several older people would come and sit in the same area and they would be taken away within minutes.

Finally, I asked the next person if I was in the correct place for a wheelchair. They asked why I needed one. I showed my boarding pass, and they looked at my face about to explode in tears (it had been a really rough few days…) and apologized.

They said that I looked young and they thought I was waiting for someone; that they had no idea. They said they are not used to anyone young and healthy-looking, sitting and waiting for a wheelchair, and they apologized again.

After I shared my story with the airline worker, she was genuinely shocked and saddened by what I had been through the past few days. She explained that she always had an image of what a person "in a wheelchair" looked like. She brought me to the gate and told me that she would no longer judge someone just by his or her age when they are sitting in a handicap area.

Not once during all the stares, judging, whispering, or disbelief did I snap back or get angry. What would that help? Isn't it better to be a beacon of light for Jesus Christ and to show others that it's okay to make mistakes and we won't bite their heads off? My feelings did get hurt and it made me sad and frustrated at times, but through it all, I knew that if God would bring me to it, He would bring me through it....

Strength in My Storm

Chapter 13
Clinical Trial?

Coming home after the funeral was such a blur. So much happened in such a short time I became overwhelmed. My heart was truly thankful that I was able to travel. However, my heart was also hurt and grieving for my mama. Add to it all, I was missing my husband and my three boys.

I hardly remember coming home. I do remember I was going to see the doctors for a follow-up that Wednesday, April 30th, so I was excited for that. I remember seeing the plastic surgeon first, and he took out the rest of my drainage tubes; that was like the best day *ever!!!* Showers were going to be so much easier without having to wear a necklace to hold all of my drainage tubes! We forget about the little things that we do every day that we take for granted – showers were one of them for me.

Then we went to see the other surgeon and she confirmed that they found cancer in three areas. They ended up finding two tumors in my left breast – one was very aggressive – and the one in my lymph nodes.

Next step – meet with the oncologist. The doctor didn't think that I would need radiation, but she would send my info off; if they needed to see me, they would contact me. I had a good feeling I wouldn't be hearing from them. I'd explain it as another "gut feeling" I had.

Then, it was finding out if I had to do chemotherapy. All I could do was stay in prayer, and let God know that no matter what happened that I knew He was with me and he would not let me go through this storm alone; that as long as I kept praising Him through everything, I could get through anything. It was a daily reminder, sometimes an hourly reminder, but I had to in order to keep calm and push the doubt and fear away.

What I did not expect and what they didn't mention was that I would be in constant pain from the expanders. During the bi-lateral mastectomy, they put in the expanders to start making room for the implants that eventually go in.

They have to "expand" the chest first. Now that I had a flat chest, with *nothing* there, I would have to go in weekly and get injections into the expanders to fill them up.

Imagine a constant pressure in your chest. Expanders are inserted behind the muscle, then push them out. It's constant pain and pressure that does not goes away until the next surgery! This is when I learned I would not sleep through the night again – at least not during this part of the reconstruction.

Things like this are what they don't tell you when you are getting your options. I had no idea that I would be in pain 24/7 for months after the surgery. I tried not to show it, but between the constant pain and the meds, you can see why my household was a mess. I kept praying that chemo would not be added onto everything else.

May 5, 2014 I met with my oncologist. He had a great sense of humor, and I knew right away he was the perfect oncologist for me! You know how crazy us Canadians can be!!

I was told I really wasn't the right category and I didn't fit "the mold" for most breast cancer patients. I still find it interesting that they would say that, as there is no "normal" for breast cancer. It happens at all ages to many body types.

I volunteered to be checked for "oncotype testing" and clinical trial. Usually this was only done in women over 50. I believe it was when there are only two areas of cancer. I was under 50 and had 3 areas with cancer. Yet, for some amazing reason, I was able to qualify! All God and prayer right there.

However, this meant yet another important decision. Would I allow myself to have my hormones synthetically controlled? What were the adverse side effects? How would I respond? What were the risks? It was not clear at the time that we had a lot more options available to us, because they weren't shared with us.

They sent the "stuff" they took out from the surgery to California to test it and see if chemotherapy would be a benefit. They tested all types of things.

Regarding analysis and testing – it's nerve racking! You go to an appointment, receive a bunch of information, get handed brochures or informational papers. Then you go get blood work or specimen samples and then… you wait.

As many tests that I did, it never became easier – I just wanted answers, results, and information! I wanted to know so that it would stop my mind from wandering.

Waiting for the "oncotype" test results was no different. I constantly checked my phone, logged in to my M.D. Anderson back office, and even called a few times to check on the status.

I was anxious because I didn't want to go through radiation or chemo, but I knew in my heart that I had to prepare myself for the worst-case scenario. Well, as soon as I had made the decision to accept the very real possibility of chemo and radiation therapy, I got another call.

By the grace of God, my test results came back and we would come to find that having chemo would not be a huge benefit and radiation was not needed. I never had one day of chemo or radiation – almost unheard of for someone with stage 2 cancer.

I was not in shock about it – I knew exactly who had planned that out and who my praise was going to….

Strength in My Storm

Chapter 14
Giving and Receiving

Without thinking about it, we judge. We judge how people look, what they may be wearing, driving, drinking, eating, or a place they may be at. Even people who are least judgmental... *judge*. Just human nature, I think. I don't even think most of us intend to.

During my journey I've been part of many people's judgments. I've learned to smile and know that they are honestly just ignorant about the situation, so why be upset, because people generally mean well. I've learned that when you are judging someone else, it's something you see in him or her that is also in you, perhaps something you have not dealt with or something you don't like about yourself.

During my storm, I tried to be very open and honest about what I've gone through since the day I found out I had breast cancer. When someone asked, I told them what I could, or what I knew. When someone was genuinely interested, I shared openly. There are many people that didn't ask and I didn't go out of my way to call and tell them what I was going through. Maybe they were afraid to; maybe it made them nervous; maybe it was too close to home for them. I don't know... and that's okay. When people genuinely wanted to know, they reached out, and to those that did, I shared.

There were times I wished people would call me and ask, or send me a private message. And there were some people who did, and that meant the world to me. But usually people just "looked" at me and since I "looked good" they thought everything was fine. Just because people look good on the outside does not mean that they are not hurting inside or just under the surface.

No journey is the same for anyone diagnosed with cancer and some people have had bad experiences with loved ones, family, friends, or even themselves. One thing I know is that if you have never actually been diagnosed with cancer, it's hard for you to truly understand.

Honestly, I feel I can say this because I had loved ones who passed away from cancer and have been diagnosed myself, so I have now seen and been on both sides. My brother passed away at age eight from Leukemia, my Baba (Dad's mom) from cancer, my dad from cancer, my mom from cancer, and two great aunts from cancer. That's a lot in one close family, and I'm not including my aunt who had breast cancer and is currently doing great, praise God!

My point is that I watched people I loved suffer with different kinds of cancer. It was hard, draining, stressful, sad… so many things. In the end, I thought I understood or had some knowledge because my mom and dad went through it and I was there. But in reality, being with someone and helping them through cancer and having been told you have it yourself is so very different, and I never would have guessed that.

The decisions you think you would make and the decisions you actually make can be so different. Like I mentioned, I would have told you before cancer that I would do everything entirely natural and I would never have a surgery.

What I prayed for and what I received, were two totally different things, yet I have complete peace knowing this was my path, even though it may not be someone else's.

So many people have judged me for my choices, because it wasn't their choice. I had people give me a hard time and actually look down on me because I decided I was doing a bi-lateral mastectomy. They told me that I should not be taking anything out that I was born with. Others told me I was wrong for taking any medications at all, and made me feel very bad about what they considered was abuse of my body.

All these people had great intentions, but each of us has our own journey and what might be for one, is not for another. The people who gave opinions had never even had cancer, but had known someone who had cancer, so they were giving me advice on something they had never even personally been through. Again I say, it's not the same knowing someone and being diagnosed yourself. I know people mean well, and that's why I have not taken personal offense to comments or judgments. However, there were many times that I would have just loved a hug or something positive to be said instead of telling me what I should be doing and what I was doing wrong.

Going through cancer can be exhausting enough and when you add everyone else's opinions on what they think you should be doing, instead of just praying for you and supporting you, it gets tiring and draining emotionally.

What I would have liked was for everyone to just stop and think before they offered up *their* opinion to someone going through a hard time or a storm. God calls each of us to a different path for His reasons so that the end result will glorify our Lord and Savior, not us.

When people look at me and ask in a confused face, "You had breast cancer? Oh, you don't look like it!" (while they immediately stare down at my chest, which makes me giggle every time!!!), I smile and say, "Yes," while knowing that cancer is not something that you can see by looking at a person.

Cancer is not on the outside. You can't pick out a person and say, "Yep, they have cancer." I have learned to take that reaction as a compliment and a chance to praise God for all the health and strength and comfort He has given me.

Every time I look in the mirror, I see the scars on my body – each time I get out of the shower, each time I get dressed. You can't see the scars after I'm dressed, but they are there and they are real; they are a reminder to me every day that I am still learning to love myself and my new body, to remember that neither the scars nor cancer define me.

That's why it's so important that I share how I feel, because most people just don't know, and I honestly believe they do mean well. If you know someone with cancer or any disease, know they hurt and they have scars, on the inside, outside, or both. They have suffered. Don't minimize it; don't judge them – just love them and let them know you are there for them.

At some point during that period, I realized that I had to take care of me so that I could take care of everyone else. That was not my usual way of being. I am the type that will make sure everyone else is fine; that everyone has enough food, and they are happy. My heart is so happy when I can do for others; it is the best, most natural feeling in the world to me. When I give, it makes me feel like I am helping someone, blessing them, making them happy. I don't even want a big thank you or anything – just seeing them smile is the joy.

However, receiving is another thing. When others tried to do for me, I wouldn't let them – I had to be the giver, I had to be the one paying, I had to be the one who still brought food when I didn't need to. I had to help with clean up or I had to watch other parents' kids at play dates so that the parents could enjoy themselves. Doing that didn't faze me – I just did it and others expected it because that's what everyone had come to know.

Being diagnosed with breast cancer, I had to learn to *stop* and let others help me. I had to let others feel the same joy of helping that I got to feel when I was being of service. Me not allowing them to help was taking their joy away, and who was I to do that?

Why did I not allow people to help me? My mom was very independent and hardly asked for help, always doing something for others. Even when she cooked, when I asked to help she wouldn't let me; everything had to be done a certain way. As they say, I guess I was a product of my environment. Watching my mom do everything on her own made me feel like I needed to be the same way, when in fact, I did not.

I had people in my life who were used to receiving from me. I was the one who freely gave my time and energy to help with their challenges. However, when the roles were reversed, some people didn't know how to take the fact that I was just not physically, mentally, or emotionally able to.

Even if I told someone or posted on social media that I was having a hard day or just had a surgery, there were still people who would call or text and want me to do something for them – and there were a few times I did. But there came a point when I had to say no. Not because I was selfish, but because I was just coping minute-by-minute myself.

This was the point where I prayed for God to show me what to do. I can't blame others for wanting me to be the person I was for the whole time they knew me – the giver – but it was a time in my life that I needed support, love, and others' blessings. And believe it or not, some people just didn't understand that.

That is something that I created with my giving nature, so I don't blame anyone but me. Watching my mom suffer and go through what she did showed me how I needed to do things differently and let people in to help me, because I knew I could not do it alone.

The people who saw this change in me and didn't understand what I needed to do for myself, I had to let go from my life. Some people slowly distanced themselves, no longer texting or calling me. That's how I knew that our season together had passed, and I was okay with it.

That doesn't mean I don't love them or I'm not thankful for having had them in my life. But when you go through a storm and you can't lean on others, they are not people to surround yourself with. Your core group is who will lift you up, encourage you, give to you, and love you no matter what.

By the end of my surgeries I was shocked at who was there for me and who wasn't; yet I also understand that God brings people in your life for different reasons and seasons, and I'm thankful for each person who has crossed my path.

Facing the diagnosis of breast cancer was life changing for me. Learning that I needed to put me and my needs first was a challenge, and still is, but I'm learning that when I don't take time for me, that I can't help others. I am a better mama when I have had quiet time, prayer time, time to write or get a pedicure – and when I ask others for help when I need it.

Chapter 15
Tamoxifen and Other Drugs

Being on a synthetic hormone such as Tamoxifen is a challenge in itself. It had been a few months and the side effects of the Tamoxifen had been horrible for me. To help with them, the doctors gave me more meds, which did not agree with me.

After spending months exhausted, passing out in the middle of the day, and having no energy for doing much of anything, I was not a fan of the meds. It is so opposite of my personality, so it was challenging for me. It was extremely hard on my boys and husband as well. I could see myself being such a different person, and it affected the whole dynamic of the house.

Some of the side effects were rage, horrible mood swings, becoming anemic, loss of memory, and more... much more. One odd side effect was that of my ears. My hearing would go in and out; my right ear would feel like it was filled with water on some days and then on other days it would be dry and crusted like psoriasis, causing major itchiness and burning. It was a vicious cycle.

I also realize now how irritated you can get from not hearing people speak. Everyone I talked to had to repeat what he or she said. I couldn't hear half the time, so people were frustrated with me or me with them and I had to have the television volume on 36! Who does that? Old people and ME!

During the week, I would drive to drop off my youngest son Dylan at his preschool, and arriving home would have no memory of where I went. That happened almost daily and it started to scare Aaron and me.

That anxiety started to affect Aaron's job. He found he could not concentrate if he knew I had to go out and drive. He would stress about me getting to my location, would I remember, would I pass out, would I be in an accident and he wouldn't know? He found himself distracted a lot because of worrying about me.

The Tamoxifen added extra hormones to my body. Now, I'm already a girl. I have hormones, but nothing too bad; I was very blessed. Then add Tamoxifen. Good gravy, hormonal freight train coming through! As much as I joke about it, I was scared of how it affected my mind and body — more than I let on.

I have never felt this way in my life. The hormones, the unexpected and out of the blue anger and rage, it actually scared me. It caused so much hormonal havoc that I could not even leave the house during my period each month, and I became anemic. I would bleed through tampons and a pad in less than 30 minutes and if I sneezed or coughed there was blood everywhere. How do you leave the house, or do anything when you can hardly walk around? What kind of life was this?

So, what did they do? Add more meds to calm me down, which caused additional side effects. I was useless between 1pm – 4pm, sometimes even longer. I wasn't sleeping at night from the pain of the expanders. I would be up at least 4-5 times a night, and sometimes could not fall back asleep for an hour.

Between not sleeping at night and the effect of the meds on my system, the couch was a place I lived on. I was lethargic, I became docile, and that goofy, fun-loving Michelle was hidden behind medication. I almost turned into a different person.

I could see it taking a toll on Aaron, whether or not he would show it or say it. There were times Aaron got short-tempered with me, because he had to repeat everything. Then he would ask me a question or tell me something and five minutes later I couldn't remember he even told me anything, and then he would turn around and I would be passed out on the couch.

My one saving grace: having daily sex. When we had sex, I felt better; I felt like a woman and I felt wanted — so I asked him daily for sex. However, the days we did not have sex became, "Why won't you have sex with me? Don't you find me attractive?"

How crazy is that? If we had sex six out of seven days that week, I felt like he didn't want me enough because that one day we didn't make out. It was all in my head – the meds were messing with my thoughts. I wouldn't normally feel or think Aaron didn't want me or wasn't attracted to me, but having these meds in my system really fogged my thoughts and my reality became skewed. Who would think that a tiny little pill could do that?

Watching the boys look at me differently and wonder why I would just sit under a blanket on the chair, I could see the concern and worry in their eyes. My oldest, Daniel, would be affected the most, as he worried right away that I would be dying if I was not getting up for hours.

One day Daniel came up to me in tears and handed me a note, which I still have. It said that he would do anything to protect me, even if he had to fight someone. He said he would die for me. The note shocked me. Why did he think he would have to do anything to protect me? He was just a child!

When I asked him, he told me he already lost Nona, he couldn't lose me. My heart was broken. This was affecting my child more than I ever thought. It made me feel guilty, ashamed that I wasn't being stronger for the family. But it also showed me the kind of love the boys had for me, and how much my state worried and hurt them.

His fear of losing his mama was evident, and even though I could see it in his eyes, I couldn't stop the effects of the meds. Where was my energy? Where was my fun-loving spirit? Where was the mama that was supposed to be taking care of *them*?

When I could muster the energy, I was up and doing more then I should because I just wanted to "feel normal." I wanted to be "the old me." So I would go, go, go, go and do everything I needed or wanted to do that I couldn't the previous few days or weeks. And every time, I would overdo it and crash – and when I crashed, I crashed hard.

I would pay for over doing it, sometimes sleeping for almost the whole day, which brought more concern to the house. Aaron would be constantly checking on me and I could see his worry.

How he was able to work through all of this amazes me to this day – what a strong man.

Due to all my bleeding, we saw an OBGYN and the options were: Mirena, which was a birth control method; ablation, where I believe they burn the entire insides of my uterus; or a hysterectomy, where they take out ALL of my insides. Really? From what we were told, hysterectomies are quite common, especially with estrogen-positive breast cancer, but current practice is to avoid the drastic measure, due to new medicine technologies.

They recommended the Mirena for me. I didn't feel at peace with any of the options. I prayed and my answer was 'not right now.' I heard horror stories about Mirena, but more than that, I didn't have that comfortable feeling in my gut, so I said no to all of the choices.

Between bleeding, the side effects of the meds, and the chaos I was causing in my house, what did I do to get through each day? I kept praying to God. I kept thanking God for each day, being grateful for each moment, and for healing me. Each day, if only for a moment, I praised God for all He had done for me and all He continued to do for me.

It may sound a bit negative describing how I was feeling, but it's really not. I'm just being honest about how the medication made me feel, how it affected me. There may be someone out there right now going through the same thing and they need to know they are not alone. This was my reality through this. Meds affect every person differently, and for me, the meds were not agreeing with my body. The reason I could get through each day was because God was and God *is* faithful in *all* things, and my strength came from Him.

There were a few very hard moments when I couldn't understand why this was happening. I thought, almost all of my surgeries are over, at least the worst of them, why this? Why was I not feeling better? I could not believe that I felt worse after surgery, after they had taken the cancer out of my body. How is that possible?

Finally, I got to see a new oncologist and she said she was going to change my meds. I was so happy!

After a couple of pity parties – okay maybe a few more than that – I was getting a change in meds! Woohoo! For each pity party, I had to stop myself. There is so much worse that I could have been going through. I could have had chemo, I could have had radiation, I could have been in a hospital, I could be dead. I had nothing to be sad about – but everything to be thankful for. It is all in the perception.

Sometimes when you are in the midst of a "storm" it's hard to see the positive and the blessings. This is when we must look even harder and find the little things for which we can thank God. That was my daily struggle and not many people knew it – finding something each day to be thankful for.

Being positive meant I had to focus on the basics – starting my day by thanking God for my sight so that I can see my boys. Thank you God for my legs so that I can stand up and walk. Thank you God for giving me another day to be with my boys and husband. I meant each word. I had to stay positive, as the meds would take control over me and send me down a dark path each day. I had to fight to stay in God's light.

Not in a million years did I think taking some medications would put me where it did. I never knew it would affect my mind, body, and spirit the way it did. Medications can really mess you up, especially if they do not agree with your body. I'm thankful my husband always made me push through and tell the doctor that something needed to change and to not settle. This is *my* body and if it doesn't feel right, then maybe that is God's way of saying, "This is not the right thing for you." It was about me realizing I had to put myself first and speak up for myself – that I was important.

Strength in My Storm

Chapter 16
No One Talks About Side Effects

The oncologist who put me on the "oncotype" moved to do research in another state. When he left, all of his patients went into "limbo" so there was no one to talk to regarding my side effects. We called several times to make an appointment with a new physician, only to be told that I wasn't assigned to a different oncologist yet. Once I was, they would let me know.

A couple of months later, after an appointment with the plastic surgeon, we went to the oncology department and told them we would not leave until we got an appointment with a new oncologist. We were told that they didn't take "walk-ins" and that I would have to call. We calmly explained that we had been calling for weeks and still had no doctor, and that the side effects were harsh and affecting me in a horrible way. Standing firm on getting an appointment before we left the building, we waited over an hour until finally, they gave us an appointment with my new doctor.

Although I was uncomfortable pressing them for an appointment, I was also not feeling heard. During that time I began to have concerns about being at that hospital. For me, it seemed that once the surgeries were over, the post-surgery patient care was subpar.

The new oncology doctor stopped my old breast cancer medication and started a new one, called Anastrozole, all within two days. That first week was rough to say the least – on my boys, my husband, and me. I learned that it takes some time for the meds to come out of your system, and in the process saw that nothing is ever easy – simple, yes – easy is another thing.

My mind was still so foggy from the medication I could hardly remember what I did an hour before, never mind the day before, and I know it was frustrating for my boys and my husband. Heck, it frustrated me like crazy! Aaron would tell me that he told me something, and I would be like... Uh, no you didn't... and in reality, he sure did. It was a daily challenge for both of us.

Overhearing Aaron talking to people a few times really was a punch in the face. I don't know if he knew I heard or not, but I know he wasn't trying to hide anything; he was just being open and honest. Both times I heard him brought me to tears.

Those few times I heard Aaron describe "me" and how the medications were affecting me, made me feel horrible. Listening to him talk to someone else about how I acted – my rage, my sadness, my pain, and my personality change – was too much for me to hear. When I overheard Aaron talk, it was like he was describing someone else, and it hurt my heart beyond what I can explain. My medications were affecting him a lot more than I realized and I felt such guilt for putting him through that.

At one point he described me as living with someone with Alzheimer's, but that he couldn't get mad because he knew it was not my fault. He said he had never seen me this bad and it broke his heart to see what the medication did to me – to my mood, my body, and my mind. Watching other people suffer because of something you can't control is the hardest thing for me, and hurt my heart the most.

Looking back, I remember being in that same position when my Papa Smurf had cancer, and watching him suffer and be in pain. That still makes my heart hurt because there was nothing that I could do for him. Then being there off and on with my mama I could see the pain she was in from her cancer, and see how the medication was changing her into someone else and I could not do a thing to help her.

Being the person watching as the person you love suffers or endures a hard time is a challenge. Now I was on the other side and Aaron had to endure the feeling of helplessness.

Even though I never wanted to feel like a burden or hurt someone like that, I knew it was out of my control. I understood it was something I had to go through to be a testimony about God and His amazing grace and love. There are times I just wish my boys or my husband did not have to be hurt in the process.

Being on the other side, I can empathize with their pain, their hurt, and their frustration and helplessness. I've been there in a small way and I prayed every day for them to have complete peace from God and strength beyond measure from Him as well.

It's funny because as I mentioned earlier, I thought after the surgeries that I was done – that is was all over. I never thought for a minute that I would feel worse afterward. No one prepared me for *post*-cancer and *post*-surgeries.

Through this, I have seen some great things. There are times God shows you why you go through things, and I think He was showing me. My mama was on Tamoxifen for her cancer. Near the end of her life she changed, her moods, the way she was, and the way she acted. The meds turned her into an easily-angered person, with mood swings that surpassed any description. She was needy and paranoid and couldn't be alone. More than anything, she lost the independence that made her strong. Being on these meds myself, I began to understand her struggle.

We knew deep down it was the medications and not Mama, but it's still so hard to see a loved one suffer or be hard and mean to you when you know they love you so much. Being on the Tamoxifen myself, I can understand more now and I do have greater compassion because I know firsthand that you honestly cannot control your thoughts or mind at times on medication.

Personally experiencing out of the blue rage and anger from something in my body that didn't belong was something that I faced every day, and the thoughts that entered my mind that I could not control *freaked me out.* There was more than one time that I felt everyone would be better off if I was dead and away from them, so that I wouldn't be a burden to them or hurt them anymore. There honestly were a few times I held a knife and said, wouldn't it be better if I just stabbed myself and left? As the words came out, the look on Aaron's face will forever be in my mind: despair, hurt, sadness, confusion, helplessness – all feelings that my words and my mouth caused him – and all reactions from the medications.

Meds can mess with you and your hormones; but it doesn't define who you are. I believe I needed to go through this so that I could show greater grace and love to others. Going through all of those emotions and losing complete control makes you either cling to God or walk away. I had to spend each minute clinging to God and relying on His strength because I could not do it alone.

As for the new breast cancer meds they put me on, they came with their new set of side effects. My head was still fogged up and now we were adding joint and muscle pain into the mix of things, along with rashes everywhere!

If you know anyone on medications and they are harsh, or different than they used to be, please show grace. They have no control over their reaction to the medication. What means the most are the friends, family, and loved ones who support them and love them and show them that they are there through it all. Encourage them to talk to their doctor to see what other choices they have; when we stand up for our bodies and ourselves, it makes a difference. And showing kindness while someone is going through a "storm" means more than words can ever say.

Chapter 17
Will My Boys be Scarred for Life?

One of the hardest things of going through breast cancer has been watching how my boys react. They were eight, five, and three at the time of my diagnosis and they have all reacted differently, yet it has affected them all deeply.

When my mom was in the last stages of her life with bone cancer I would talk to my boys about how "Nona" had cancer, she was sick and getting weaker, to try and prepare them for when she did pass away.

They were used to talking to my mom a couple of times a week, so when they would no longer hear her voice and talk to her, it was hard for them to understand why.

When we sat down and told the boys that I had breast cancer, they had a few questions; not many, as I'm sure it was sinking in and they didn't quite understand. Over the months to follow, it became harder and harder.

A couple of days after Nona passed away, we told the boys. My middle son David cried uncontrollably. I was taken aback at how he reacted. My oldest son Daniel was very sad; he had been very, very close to Nona and I can tell it still affects him to this day. Dylan didn't really understand, but in the months to come, he showed it in his own way by being clingy and being sad when I would leave, and wrap his arms around my neck and say, "Don't go, Mama."

After telling the boys, bedtimes were hard. Each night, they would pray for me to feel better and for Nona to feel better and pray that I wouldn't die from cancer too. They prayed for Nona to come back and I would explain again that Nona had passed away and that they would see her again one day in heaven.

That would just cause more heartache, and I would break down with them in tears. Everything was just too fresh for me. I just had surgery and I felt so different with no breasts.

My mama, who I called for *everything* daily was gone and I was not going to hear her voice anymore. I would randomly call her and ask about a recipe or ask about something I saw and she always had the answer. I was not going to be able to ask advice and I was not going to be able to tell her how much I loved her. The boys felt the same way.

Each bedtime became, 'please Lord don't let my mama die from cancer.' Each time they prayed it, it broke my heart and I cried. Then they would ask me, "If Nona died from cancer, will you die from cancer?"

We would assure them that I was not going anywhere, that God had a plan for me and that I would be there to see their weddings and their children. Every night they asked the same thing, and every night I would give the same answer to try and reassure them.

They would squeeze my neck so tight, and they would say, "I don't want to let you go, Mama; I don't want you to die." Even writing this, it brings tears. I can still hear their tiny little voices. They have such sweet hearts and I can't imagine the pain they were going through at such a young age.

At one point my middle son David blocked it out that my mom had passed away and then he prayed for her to feel better one night and I had to explain again that she had passed away.

He innocently asked, "So, I will never get to see her again when we go up there?" (meaning in Canada when we visit). I explained that he wouldn't – to which he broke down all over again, breaking my heart again. The two of us cried together and hugged for a long time. Losing my mom was hard for all of us, since she was an active part in our lives.

Those nights I would take the extra time and snuggle them, kiss them, and pray with them and let them know that I was there for them and that I would be for a long time.

What is the hardest part of being diagnosed with breast cancer? The affect it has had on my children. They were so young and didn't quite understand.

Even when my allergies acted up and I was down on the couch, right away, the boys changed their demeanor and asked, "Are you sick? Are you okay? What can we do?" They want to snuggle me and lay beside me. I try not to even use the word "sick" anymore because that word has scared them – I see it in their eyes.

The good thing is that they see Mama is strong, Mama has a powerful and amazing Lord Jesus Christ who strengthens her, and their Mama never gives up. I hope that as time goes by, that is what they continue to see and the fear goes away along with the hurt.

Strength in My Storm

Chapter 18
Another Change – Moving AGAIN

After renting a home in Katy, Texas for six months, with everything going on we decided it might be time to find a home. With my first surgery over and knowing there would be more to come, we really wanted to settle in and make a home for the boys. On Canada Day, July 1, 2014, we bought a home in Grayson Lakes – the best subdivision *ever!*

We packed everything up and rented a U-Haul for the day, then moved everything ourselves, meaning Aaron did all the heavy lifting as I packed. Here was the amazing thing: Aaron had just started at his new job in December, only seven months before, yet people from his work were there, ready to help.

As everything was getting packed, Aaron was arranging to take the carpet out of the new house because I have allergies – well, when he got to the house, his coworkers had already ripped up the carpet and underpad.

My heart was so touched. As it was, this was the second time we were moving in seven months, the boys had just experienced their mom go through surgery, they were still dealing with their Nona passing away, and here was another change, which meant their third school in a year. That's a lot for anyone to take, especially children.

Our "hood" had an annual 4th of July parade and party; America is crazy for their celebrations and I love it! So a big parade came by our house and the neighbors told us to go to the clubhouse for food and swimming, so we did!

There, we met some families, and one mom, Kara, told me about this playgroup and that there was a Bunco night coming up.

Looking back at it, I see God putting me exactly where I needed to be. This was a group of ladies that I needed to meet.

As uncomfortable as I was about going to a Bunco night alone and not knowing a soul, I bucked up and thought to myself, 'you can do this, you can!' I was self-conscious about my chest, as the expanders were still in, even though my chest size was just about the same as it used to be. But it was hard as rocks, uncomfortable, and big. No one there would know the difference, but I felt that difference every day.

I went to Bunco and it was fun. I made a point to try and chat with people. I was drawn to one girl, Stephanie. There was something about her heart that stood out to me right away. She had a kind smile, she was genuinely interested in getting to know me, and as many of the other girls were chatting openly, you could tell they had long time friendships that perhaps she didn't. She was super-tall, thin and beautiful, with a good sense of humor, which I liked. We stood at the end of the kitchen counter chatting and getting to know each other, and I could tell right away we would be friends.

After Bunco, we all went outside and talked, and at that point I shared that I had breast cancer and that I just had surgery a couple of months before. The ladies were shocked, but not as much as I was that I shared that the first time I met them. I knew that if I was going through this, then I had to be open and vulnerable and share my story to everyone I met.

After I shared, one of the ladies, Audrey, said that our husbands worked together. Her hubby had come to help at the house. I told her how thankful we were for them.

It was these ladies who would set up meals for me for each surgery I had and would check on me, pray for me, and support me. All of these ladies from the "hood" became friends, and again I got to see God's hand at work.

Without me being brave and accepting an invitation, doing the uncomfortable and going and walking through the door that God opened, I would not have had the blessings I did from all of these wonderful ladies. They were a huge part of teaching me how to receive.

Chapter 19
Reconstruction

September 8th came quick… kind of! Pre-op day arrived and oddly enough I was excited about this next part… the reconstruction. My sister Julie flew in from Thunder Bay, Canada the night before. She was staying with my youngest, Dylan, so I relaxed, knowing she was with him.

Julie coming here allowed Aaron and me to go to the pre-op together and for him to be at the hospital with me all day for surgery. I also knew my kids would love extra time with Aunty Ju Ju Bean!

Pre-op went great and I asked *a lot* of questions, none of which I can remember now – funny how that is. We want to ask all these questions and know all these facts "just in case" so we know what will happen. But after the surgery, and everything went great, I completely forgot what I had asked. Maybe that's me, or a side effect of the meds; either way, I was happy to forget that time!

At the hospital I was so calm and relaxed, almost oddly so. The week before I had suffered terribly with allergies, so bad it was almost like I had the flu. I couldn't swallow, my throat was swollen, and I could not breathe through my nose at all. The Friday before I had to ask Aaron to come home from work because I was freaked out that I needed to rest and get rid of this before my surgery!

If I couldn't breathe, how could they do a surgery and put the tube down my throat when I went under. I worried for days, and then Aaron ministered healing to me and I remembered where *all* my burdens are *supposed* to go – to Jesus Christ. That's when I finally calmed down again and felt God's perfect peace. My control and trust issues were rearing their ugly head again. That is how easily fear and control can creep back.

That day at pre-op I had to get the regular blood and urine tests, and once I got to the anesthesiologist they said my throat looked good (thank the *Lord!*) and that my hemoglobin was low by one point, which I felt was a side effect of the meds.

After the day at the hospital, I came home and got the "green light" and when I called in at 5:00 pm to see what time my surgery was, I found out I was the first one – YAY! That meant I had to be there at 5:30 am. Again, I didn't mind, because the earlier I got in, the earlier I would get out and be home for supper!

No one could believe this reconstruction would be a day surgery, but it was. They would be taking out my expanders, putting in the silicone implants, then grafting material from my tummy to fix around the breast. Because the area was so swollen, they also did liposuction on my sides, almost under my armpit, where the tubes were inserted for the first surgery. (I totally should've asked for liposuction on my love handles... dang it!!!)

Seemed like a lot to do for a day surgery, but I trusted my doctor and my Lord Jesus Christ, who gave me complete peace and made me feel that each step of the way I was choosing the correct path. What mattered to me was that I would glorify and honor *Him* in all things.

Well, I was ready for surgery, knowing that I could handle it because I had put all my faith and trust in God and that I had so many wonderful friends and family praying for me. My friend Stephanie had suggested setting up a meal train for me with the neighborhood girls, and they also offered prayers, which was exactly what we needed. In case you don't know, a meal train is the best thing since sliced bread! You create it online and you can include anyone to sign up to bring meals to people in need. It really was a lifesaver for our family and I was so thankful for it.

Prayer is so powerful and I can honestly say that I could feel it, since the peace I felt that morning going into surgery is not natural; it really is God's perfect peace.

September 9th, 2014 at 4:30am came early to leave our home to get to M.D. Anderson for my breast reconstruction surgery, that's for sure! The drive to the hospital was very calm, with a prayer and then our usual joking around and making light and fun in the moment. We got to M.D. Anderson, and checked in at the Mays Clinic.

They called me in and I thought it was just for weight and blood pressure, since they told Aaron to wait, so I didn't think much of it. They took me back to my "room" and asked me to get dressed – or should I say undressed – for surgery, including putting on my cool socks with no toes… those are pretty fun to put on! I sat there and for a moment I panicked, wondering why Aaron was not back there, why I was already changing and he wasn't in the room, and if they were going to let him in. There was that nasty fear poking its head in again.

In a matter of minutes, I went from calm and peaceful to freaking out because I didn't want anyone giving me instructions without Aaron there. I didn't trust my memory or my thoughts and I had nothing to write with. What if it was important info? What if they were telling me about possible complications? What if? My head started spinning.…

Then I stopped. I smiled and remembered all that God had already done for me. Where He had placed me, how He had made my paths VERY clear and how He had been with me every step of the way; I was not alone. I was immediately calm and in His perfect peace once again. I could feel all the prayers of friends and family, and it was just amazing!

I got into my "bed" and a chaplain walked by and asked me a few questions and then we said a prayer together and I was full of smiles! Then I was back to my old self, telling jokes with the nurse and just being happy and thankful for all I had. Aaron came in and I felt complete. God is good, all the time.

The poor nurse in training struggled to get my IV in and took quite a few times, but I sat quietly and told her it was no problem. Did it hurt? YEP! Would me complaining help anything? NOPE. So why complain? She needed encouragement, not a grumpy patient! So I laid there as still as I could remembering not to let that nasty control creep back in.

The rest is a blank until I woke up in recovery. All was good, the surgery was a success and there was my husband waiting there for me with a smile.

Strength in My Storm

Chapter 20
Tell the Truth

Going to the oncologist January 21st made me a bit anxious. My medications were still giving me pretty harsh side effects, and I kept praying for real clarity on what to do. All I kept getting from God when I prayed was to wait until the appointment, and to be honest about how I felt.

A big struggle for me is telling anyone, especially doctors, exactly how I'm feeling, and being able to put myself first. I like to just shrug things off as "I'm fine" and "I'm doing great, could be worse" because in fact, I am fine and things could be worse.

Feeling like I am a burden to people will cause me to not share things with them so that I don't worry them. I didn't even want to think for a second that the meds would get the best of me, so I tried to ignore it. Kind of funny to try and ignore some of my side effects, but I was doing my best to not give full disclosure. Yet in reality, they were affecting me, and everyone around me.

I have learned with breast cancer, you have to keep a list and inform the doctor of *all* the side effects, since this is how they can monitor you, the meds, and if they have to look for anything else. I started being brutally honest with the doctors about exactly how I was feeling, and to tell the truth to friends when they asked.

When we went to meet with the oncologist on that Wednesday, she asked what was happening, and I pulled out my list. I guess I'm that small percentile person that has all the side effects you hear about on the commercials. You know, they play those ads for a medication and at the end it lists about 20-30 side effects really quickly! That's me – *I'm Super Special!*

At one point I told her I have uncontrollable chills, day and night. She was intrigued by the fact I had chills! She said, "Usually people get hot flashes; I have never heard of anyone getting chills." Yep, that's me, unique Michelle! For those of you who know me, you know I'm a human heater and wear shorts all year round even when I lived in Canada, so for me to be cold is unknown territory.

We took out one of the medications for a trial because it was doing more harm than good. They decided to change out Anastrozole for Zoladex for the time being, and would monitor my estrogen. The Zoladex would be a monthly infusion shot in my tummy and they thought it would help with some of the side effects I had with the daily pills.

This was just another step in my journey. I wanted to see if this would help and if my side effects would go away. There are always other paths to take. However, at that time I felt I was still on the right path where I needed to be.

Some of my side effects included blurred vision, dizziness, nausea, bone pains, muscle aches, forgetfulness (that's a polite way to put it), and of course my hearing, grogginess, and seeing stars... yes, stars. Because of that, she said we should do a head scan/MRI to make sure everything was fine. Then, after telling her more side effects, like my head hurting sometimes, the out of the blue rage and anger, and the roller coaster ride of emotions, she also ordered a bone scan.

When I say more side effects, there were so many I can't even list them all because I can't even remember them all. Lots were scary, like the feelings of worthlessness and depression that crept in. Some of these feelings happened on a daily basis, if even for just a few minutes.

The logical part of me understood the need for new tests. I would rather they check everything and make sure it's just side effects from the medication and nothing else. Then there was the other part of me. My dad passed away after the cancer he had in his bones spread and went to his brain. My mom had just passed away the year before from bone cancer, and my brother Steven had also passed. Can you guess where my head went? Yep! Was I next? Did I have bone cancer? How did it spread? Was it the medication? Was it hereditary? What would I do?

I stayed strong in the office, even though I was ready to break down and cry just from the memories of what those two tests represented with my parents – death.

Could all of these symptoms be from side effects of medications that these doctors put me on, or was it something else? Once again fear crept in that they would find more cancer.

Within the week, I received the call – all was clear, all the side effects were from the meds. *Wow!*

Strength in My Storm

Chapter 21
Surround Yourself with Positive

Have you ever heard that story about the crabs in the bucket? When you put one crab in a bucket, he will try and get out. If you put more than one crab in a bucket, you don't need a lid, because the other crabs won't let the others get out – they will pull them back in!

The same is true about your life. If you don't surround yourself with people, family, and friends who want to see you succeed, they will pull you down, try and squash your dreams, and make you feel like it's too hard, it can't be done, or that you are better off where you currently are. Do not stay near those people! Get away quickly!

I have found that when I surround myself with people who are successful, that push me to be a better version of myself, people who help me dream bigger, I am a happier person! I want to be encouraged to excel at whatever I do, whether it's being a stay-at-home mom, a business owner, or an entrepreneur, I believe we can have everything we want in life if we have a goal, write it down, and then do action steps to get it.

One thing I did is put positive bible verses or sayings all around my house and on my bathroom mirror where I looked every day. When I am so filled with positive all around it causes me to smile and believe that *I can* do it.

Having a positive attitude was half the battle for me. I chose to be happy and positive during my surgeries and during recovery. I chose to be smiling at every appointment, even when my hands were shaking and my heart was trembling in fear.

While going through my storm, I chose to be around positive people who lifted me up, because it was the one time in my life that

I needed to lean on God and other people, not be the one supporting others – and I had to learn that was okay for me to do.

I learned that when I wake up with a grateful, thankful heart and start the day with prayer, the negative had a harder time creeping and sneaking in. I would literally stop and look around to see the beauty all around me, including my boys, and when I did that with a genuine heart, it was hard not to smile. Being positive really does change how you see the world and how others see you.

Another thing that helped keep me positive in my healing was starting Occupational Therapy (OT) after my surgeries. During surgeries they have to pin down your arms, so if it's a long surgery, there can be problems with straightening your arms and having full range of movement over your head.

My plastic surgeon recommended I go to OT right away to make sure there was no long-term damage. I went to Spero Rehab, where I found positive, encouraging people. I spent months in therapy, and when I was done, I had full range of motion and had begun to rebuild my muscles. Although I'm still building my strength, having therapy start so soon after my surgery really aided my healing; it was such a blessing.

Being around encouraging people gave me more confidence. The people at Spero Rehab loved hearing about my story and were always engaging and asking me questions. They cared, and that really lifted me up.

Chapter 22
Am I a Burden?

The past two years have been full of so much emotion, and Aaron has been such a rock through it all, that even he eventually needed a "what the heck" moment! Considering all that Aaron had endured putting up with the meds and their effect on me, I'm surprised he never freaked out more.

One time I remember him telling me how frustrated he was with me, that living with me was exhausting and hard, and that he couldn't even have a conversation with me because I wouldn't remember it; that my "rage sessions" may not be anything that I remember, but that my words hurt and cut him deep.

He was holding resentment and anger toward me; I could see it in his eyes. I tried explaining that I couldn't help it, that I didn't mean to – but that did not help. Words hurt. My actions hurt. As much as he showed me love, he vented and let me have it, and part of me thought I deserved it and the other part of me thought I didn't.

I didn't choose to have cancer and go through this; I was doing the best I could. But that does not mean there were no victims in the crossfire of what the meds were doing to me. How I hurt others is still the hardest part of going through this.

It is hard being with someone going through cancer, or any hard time. It's very draining and emotionally difficult because you really do not have any control. And that's hard for anyone, especially a man. All he wanted to do was fix the situation and me, and the fact that he couldn't drove him crazy.

There are so many times that I felt like a burden, and that my family and friends have had to put up with so much because of me. Between the surgeries, the past medications, reconstruction, and the meds I was on, it seemed almost never ending. There were days when I felt like I was just a burden, and I wished they didn't have to suffer because of me. Those were the days I prayed even more, because I knew it was the devil trying to take my joy, take my promises, and take my belief or faith. I have had to stop and realize that every day, every minute has been part of *my* journey, part of *my* road, and part of what is growing me closer to my Lord Jesus Christ.

When I was feeling most like a burden is when I should have written in my blog to get it out. I should have reached out more to friends and shared what I was feeling. I should have told Aaron how out of control I felt. The more you say it and put it out there, the less power the enemy has over you. I know that; I just didn't do it.

February has become a month full of mixed emotions for me. It was the month of my diagnosis, when the words "you have breast cancer" were said to me. Valentine's Day is also in February and it is a time for Aaron and I to spend time together on a date. It is also the month before my birthday.

Februarys are different now. They cause more emotion, because it marks the start of the exhaustion, the hurt, the pain, the loss, the difficulties, the stress, the worry and anxiety of the cancer journey I've been on.

And so my goal has been to start embracing the month of February and treat it differently. Now I look at February as the month that made me a stronger woman; that has changed me from the inside out. February is the month that taught me to show even more empathy toward people; that taught me that everyone is going through a struggle, whether I see it or not, and that I have the power to change people's lives by being kind and showing love and not judging others.

February is the month that I realized even more how important my family is and how important it is to have good friends by your side that you can trust and that will love you through everything – even the darkest of times, not just when it's convenient for them.

So, I've realized that February is really a month of joy – a month that I needed for me to grow and become a better person and have a closer walk with God and to learn to put *every* little worry, doubt, care, anxious thought, fear, control, *anything* at His cross, for it's not mine to bear.

For His word says, my yolk is easy and my burden is light. So why do I keep insisting on trying to carry it myself? Because I'm human.

So here I am giving it to you God. I am not a burden. I am a child of the one true King and I am thankful for every blessing in my life – including my cancer free health.

Strength in My Storm

.

Chapter 23
Laughter is the Best Medicine

Surrounding yourself with people who make you smile, is soooo important when you are going through any storm! I believe a majority of the reason I handled everything so well was because of my husband Aaron and his insane ability to make me smile in any situation. Just ask him when you see him about the naked fat man dance! HILARIOUS!!! Hee hee!

Okay, even the name of that seems odd doesn't it! On some of my harder days when I was either mourning my mom or in pain from the expanders or just exhausted from not sleeping in months, Aaron went to extreme measures to get me to smile.

He would wear his underwear, and for extra laughs he would put another pair on his head, then he would dance around the room, particularly in front of me until I would smile!

Sometimes he would play music in the background and keep dancing around and even the boys would join him on occasion, wearing underwear on their heads as well! How can that not make you smile!!

Some days he would see me getting down and say – you better smile or I'll do the naked fat man dance! Still not sure why he called it that as he is not fat at all, but it's one of my favorite dances ever!

When we would go to our weekly appointments at M.D. Anderson, he would dress up, he would ask me to dress up and do my hair, and we would make it like a date day – I loved that. Who doesn't feel better when they are all dressed up! I know I felt better. He would hold my hand, tell me jokes, make me laugh, and I would almost forget where I was… almost.

Being at a hospital like M.D. Anderson, or any cancer center, is emotional. Everywhere you look, you see people who are going through treatments, who are sad, who are alone with no support, and you see people who just had their world rocked by being told they have cancer. You can't go to a place like that without a positive mindset and unwavering faith. They are also not places you should go alone. If you have someone close to come with you, whether it's a spouse, family, or friend, bring them with you.

Those were some of the hardest and most emotional days of my journey – being at the hospital and seeing the people that sat alone, with no support and looking so lonely. Aaron and I would talk to people, and do our best to make others smile. However, there were some I know we could not reach, although they were longing for someone to support them and be there for them. For those people I would sit and pray in the quietness of my heart that they would get their strength and joy from God.

In the waiting room, Aaron and I would take selfies and kiss and some people would look at us like we were crazy, and others would smile and thank us for bringing joy to their day. Can you picture us? A young couple (by M.D. Anderson standards, since Aaron was only 33) coming in all dressed up, smiling, holding hands, joking, kissing, and taking selfies in the waiting room. We did it for us, not to offend anyone or bother anyone; we did it to stay positive, to make it a happy experience.

At the hospital, I still remember the cutest older couple telling us that watching us made their whole day. You could see the love from Aaron, as he did this to make me smile; that filled my heart so full, I can't tell you.

When we would check in at M.D. Anderson, they always asked for my medical record number, never my name (which I was not a fan of) and Aaron would always pipe up and say 1-800-HOT-MAMA! Hard not to start laughing when he did that – and most of the administrators laughed… most of them. Some people have no sense of ha ha!

I believe to work in a medical facility that deals with life changing situations, like cancer, that you should have some sort of soothing and happy demeanor. When you are at a place like M.D.

Anderson, as a patient or a caregiver, you need positive encouragement and kindness during a stressful situation.

There were those few times when we checked in that the receptionist was cold and unfriendly. I would try and make them smile and they were like statues. That would piss Aaron off like crazy – he wanted to tell them to put a bracelet on and go sit out there amongst the patients and see what it's like to sit there for hours on end waiting. Or being told you cannot leave the floor or you'll miss your appointment, so you get so hungry that you are nauseous and your hunger pains immobilize you. Or being referred to by a patient number and not your name at every appointment and being made to feel like you are more of an inconvenience and not like a human.

Some places treat the cancer, but not the patient. The cancer or any sickness will always win unless the patient feels empowered!

There were other times I went into appointments alone. When I was not being "entertained" by Aaron, I did not make a point of dressing up. I was not laughing at those appointments, and they were very different, much more challenging. Those monthly appointments when I had to go alone to get my Zoladex injections were difficult for me. When you walk into any cancer center, there is a reality of what these people are going through. You always want to have someone with you who will strengthen you and make you smile and lift you up. Not having Aaron with me at those appointments was harder than I told him; I should have been more honest and asked him to come, or asked someone to come. I know that if I would have, someone would have; again it was my lack of accepting help and receiving from others.

There is no value I can put on laughing and happiness and joy during a difficult time. I know that during my time going through my storm, it was the laughter and joy that kept me sane and helped me remember that I had so much to be thankful for.

Strength in My Storm

Chapter 24
Caregivers are Under-Rated

When my Papa Smurf was in the hospital with cancer, the three of us kids would take turns being with him, but I wasn't an actual caregiver. The nurses actually did all of the work. I didn't do much but chat with him, snuggle him, watch some sports on television with him, and love on him. Watching him suffer was hard, and let me tell you he was the best patient in the world! He made jokes to everyone, tried to make the nurses and doctors smile, and he had a joy about him that made people want to be around him. He was an amazing father whom I respected and looked up to.

Not having to be there 24 hours a day doing everything for him, as an actual caregiver does, means I really don't know what it's like to be a caregiver. I just know how it feels to watch someone you love suffer and you can't do anything to help him or her... except pray.

So many people have reached out to Aaron and I and prayed for me and asked what they could do for me. But it was very rare for anyone to ask Aaron how he was and how he might need help. There were times I even reached out to a couple of people to say that Aaron needed someone to talk to, but nothing came of it.

People don't see the effect on the caregiver and all they do. They have the brunt of the work – the pain that no one sees, the frustration, anger, and even resentment for having to take care of someone they love while watching them turn into someone they don't even know because of side effects of medication.

Marriages are broken up from diseases and trials because the caregiver is never thought of or taken into consideration for all they have to endure. I know that Aaron has endured more than his share. He has had to watch me go from his Michelle to someone who would be docile, then lethargic, with rage, and anger, crying and emotional, who could hardly get up and walk, who slept all day, closed off, then swung to being happy – and after rage fits happened I would have no memory of it. But the effects of my words or actions would last on him.

One time I started freaking out for no reason... again. I think there were some crumbs on the floor by the table where they were eating. CRUMBS! I yelled. I was crying, and I said I would be better off dead; that way no one would have to worry about me or put up with me and I wouldn't be a burden to anyone anymore. I think I said something about being better off gone, period, and that I should just leave and get out of their lives so they could be happy. *Who says those things!* Then I would storm into my bedroom, slam the door, and cry in my closet until I calmed down. Then there was the aftermath of my actions and my words... and total shame on my part for what I did once again.

Even writing about it to share with others, is embarrassing; but I want to share so that anyone else who may go through this knows they are not alone and it will get better.

If you know of someone that is the caregiver, of someone who is sick, or someone who had a stroke, or whatever it is – ask them how THEY are doing. They need to talk; they need to vent and share. They need your love and support.

They are going through as much of a hard time as the one they are taking care of and they need love, prayers, and comfort – if not more. They need the strength to get through another day without taking things personally, and having compassion to get through all they deal with.

To all of you caregivers out there, you are amazing and wonderful, and you are appreciated.

Chapter 25
Through Thick & Thin

Cancer is a lot for most people to deal with. I hear stories of people who leave their spouse after breast cancer. That the man leaves his wife because it's just too much to bear, or that he is just not strong enough to be her rock during all that will ensue. There's a lot that takes place once you are told you have cancer – more than a lot of people realize and more than people want to know. From my experience alone, I can see how divorce could happen.

You don't just get diagnosed, have a surgery, and it's done; there's just so much more. So why do people leave? I believe when the man leaves, he just feels helpless. The man is the one who likes to solve everything, he wants to fix it, make it better; and when he can't, it's hard to handle.

My belief is that they think it's something that has to do with their "manliness," when in fact it does not. They may not want to see their wife change or become different looking, which may be vain; but it's so true.

Why would the woman leave? Totally different reasons, but that happens as well. I would have a hard time leaving, as I married for better or worse, but it happens. After being on both sides of cancer, I can honestly say it's harder being on the side of watching someone going through cancer.

When you are watching a loved one with cancer, you feel helpless. You can't do anything, other than pray. You can love them, be there for them, and encourage them, but you can't take away the pain, the hurt, the suffering, or the side effects of the cancer or the medications.

When people tell me, I'm "different" than before my cancer, it hurts my heart. Inside, I feel like the same person. I love the same,

I have the same passions. I am Michelle Perzan. Others see it differently. They saw I was not as active. I hardly went out, because I was recovering. I didn't text regularly or call, because I didn't have the strength all the time to do that. So some friends called me different, because I wasn't reaching out the way I normally did, and Aaron called me different because he saw how my words and energy were totally different.

My boys saw a mama who got frustrated quicker, who blew up for socks in the living room, or someone who screamed because of something small, like crumbs on the floor. Even as that happened, the other Michelle was still in there.

Seeing my boys' eyes well up with tears, asking if I'm okay, broke my heart. There were times that I was not the strong supporter to Aaron that I should have been, instead making him feel like he failed. I did not do my job of lifting him up as his wife.

There are those glimpses I get where I have huge compassion for why people leave. It's hard. It's a struggle. I am not here to judge any man or woman who has left someone who had cancer. Until you have been put in those shoes, you don't know what you will do. I have also learned that when you try and do it yourself you will fail – to get through each day, you need to lean on God.

Do I also think that anything worthwhile is hard? *Yes.* Do I believe with my whole heart that with every struggle, hardship, or trial there comes learning, growth, and positivity? I honestly do.

Do I also believe that if we just completely trust in God that *He will* bring us through it and use our experience to help others and to glorify Him? Yes. Do I also think that this is the enemy's way of trying to attack my family and me, to try and get us to believe we are better off apart? Yes.

I believe in my heart that every part of our life is planned, better than we could ever imagine by the Author and Finisher of our faith. I know that days will be hard and there will be struggles, and if I can just keep my eyes on God and hold on to His promises for me, that I can make it to the next day.

In these dark times, that's when I know I need to cling to God the most, because He will bring me out of it and will provide ways for me to take those dark times and encourage others.

Honestly, I believe that all of these struggles will help my boys learn compassion, love, understanding, and faith. They are being shown humbleness; when I mess up, I go and apologize to them and tell them that I am sorry. It is so important to be open and honest with your children.

As dark as days can get, the sun always comes out and I am able to see God's unfailing love in my life by my church, friends, and family. There are a handful of people who know the true day-to-day struggle, but many really don't want to know. For those who don't want or need to know details, prayers are welcome, and make a difference.

There are also some people who I thought would support me through it all who haven't, and that's okay; I'm not upset. Maybe it was too hard for them, or maybe it was something else; I don't know. What I do know is that God will put people in your life that you need who will encourage you, lift you up, and support you for times you need, and He has certainly done that.

The people who truly want to see you succeed and can put you first and really want the best for you will always be there for you to encourage you, support you, and love you through your storm. Whether I am giving or receiving, my true friends are there for me like I am for them, in good times and in trying times.

Do I want to go back to being the old Michelle? To be honest, not really. Having breast cancer has made me do things I never would have. I have stepped up to speak for the Ambitious Women's Success Club, for my company Ambit Energy; I joined Toastmasters and Business Networking International (BNI), and have loved it. I co-authored the bestselling Amazon book, *Emerge: Real Stories of Courage and Truth* in September 2015. I signed up to become a John Maxwell speaker, trainer, and coach; I became an Ambitious Women's Success Club Ambassador, and I just became involved in another business in a ground floor opportunity – all since being diagnosed with breast cancer.

These are all things I would never have done, since I never had the confidence. God saw me different and so did Aaron. I believe that I have gone through what I did so that I could give back to others, so that I could encourage others and serve them. I will *not* stop talking about how God has blessed me and has given me all of these opportunities to share with others and to tell my story, because God deserves all the glory.

There are days it's hard to be a "different" Michelle because of what the meds and surgeries have done to my memory and my body. I try not to focus on that since I know I won't be that way forever.

God already took care of it; I just needed to keep walking in that faith and trust in Him. So each day I became more aware of how I used my words and how I talked to my boys and my husband.

My goal is always to be an encourager, first in my home, and then to others. I stay positive so the enemy will not be able to creep in with lies, making me think that I should ever be anywhere than where I am – part of MAD3 (our family nickname – Michelle, Aaron, Daniel, David and Dylan!).

Chapter 26
Getting Out of My Comfort Zone

When does true growth happen? When you get out of your comfort zone! This has been part of my personal development since I started working with my coach Amy Applebaum. It's funny – the more comfortable you get with something, the more you have to push yourself again to get out of your comfort zone.

For example, before my coaching, I couldn't even speak at Toastmasters without holding a copy of my speech and reading it off the paper while standing behind the lectern. Each speech I gave I began to write less on my paper and move from behind the lectern, until finally I could stand without notes and walk back and forth in front of the room.

This helped me so much in my journey, since my speeches all revolved around my breast cancer. I was able to write about it, share it, and be open and vulnerable with others.

Getting out of my comfort zone took practice; once I could do one small thing, I had to get out of my comfort zone and push myself further – that's how we all grow, by persevering and pushing ourselves to be more and do more so others can be blessed by our actions.

My husband and I set some major goals, which included us starting our own business presentation for our company, so we stepped out and did it. That made us push ourselves to actively work our business and talk to more people to fill up the room. That scared me – but I did it anyway, because I wanted to grow my business and reach out to more people. That was more important to me than the fear. My goal to bless my boys, my sister, and our family was stronger than my fear.

We already talked about fear and what it is — so why give in to it — it's false and it's not of God. Fear will be there and will creep in with everything we do — it's about recognizing it, seeing it, and doing it anyway. That's a great lesson my coach Amy Applebaum teaches me over and over and over again.

Each time I have faced my fears, I have felt so free, like I broke the chains and the stronghold over me. When you go forward in spite of your fears, that's when you grow and God shines His light on you. That's when the blessings flow because you are doing things for His glory and honor, not your own.

If you are looking to change something or you feel stuck or weighed down, get out of your comfort zone, look fear in the face, tell that lie that you have the victory in Christ, and do it — you will see your life change, and those chains and burdens you have will be broken and you will be free. In Jesus' name I pray… Amen.

Chapter 27
Second Opinions

I would never have thought I would put obedience and cancer in the same sentence. However, that is what it has been in my case. Through my whole journey of breast cancer, I have found that when I place my complete trust in God, let go of my need for control, and be a yielded vessel through obedience, that I am blessed beyond words. It is through nothing I have been able to do on my own, that's for sure, as I am a person who wants things done now, fix it quick, how can I have it immediately? I have learned and continue to learn that it's never in my timing, but only in God's divine timing. Believe me, His ways will *mind blow* what you think you want. I've learned that many times over.

Deep down, I also knew that I was in the right place at the right time that God provided for me. God provided a way for me to be at M.D. Anderson when I needed it, and I am so thankful for that and everyone God has put in my path so far, since I know my journey is not quite over.

Having prayed for months for there to be a door open for a holistic doctor or a hospital that would do some tests, I was hopeful something would happen soon. I had asked many questions at my appointments because of the horrible side effects I had been having, only to be told "there is nothing else we can do for you…." We asked for some other options, but none were given. They said I had no other options.

That's a hard statement to hear when you are not feeling like yourself, and you are putting a shot in yourself monthly that is making you feel like another person. I also knew that in God's amazing timing, a door would open, if I would just put my faith and trust in Him and be obedient.

In January 2016 I had one of the worst weeks for side effects. Even though I was on a Zoladex shot, which puts you into a menopausal state, I got my period. And I'm not talking a normal period. It came back with a vengeance. Within 24 hours I could tell I was anemic again from all of the bleeding.

Quickly, I emailed M.D. Anderson and let them know my side effects, to which the reply was – well that shouldn't be happening – contact the OBGYN. I emailed the same message to them, to which they replied the same – it shouldn't be happening. *No shit Sherlock!* I could tell you that! They said they wanted to get me in for an ultra sound and some tests – they would see me in a few weeks. A few weeks!

How lovely that was – so I would just bleed to exhaustion because my side effects were not important enough to get me in right away.

It was bad enough that when we went in for the last appointment in January, we asked again for other options and the response was, "You don't have any other options. You are going to have to tough it out for another four and a half years!" Say what? As if I, as if we, hadn't been through enough that they had the cheek to basically tell me, "Suck It Up Buttercup!"

Protocol for breast cancer patients is a five-year hormone treatment plan. I had been on meds for six months, so I had a long way to go – it didn't look too bright from where I was sitting.

Needless to say all the answers were unacceptable. Aaron was frustrated that they spoke to us like that, and after emails back and forth, filed a complaint. The lady thanked him, but Aaron's response was, "Don't thank me. If you were a patient would you want to be treated like that?"

Aaron went on a mission. He sat down and dug deep and started making calls and doing all kinds of research again. This time, Cancer Treatment Centers of America (CTCA) popped up. Amazing how that happens isn't it?

He filled out forms, and within 12 hours he was on the phone with them. In less than 24 hours, they had an appointment for me.

They wanted to see why my hormones were high, and respond to all of my side effects that I had going on. Seeing it all take place in 24 hours showed me it was all God – there was no other explanation to have it all happen so quickly, and for them to take care of everything.

CTCA paid for our flight up to Chicago, they paid for our hotel, and they paid for my three meals a day. Aaron only had to pay about 20% of the cost of his meals. I was in shock over the amazing treatment.

Was there a part of me that was nervous and a bit anxious? Yes. I would have to take a whole bunch of tests again, and that felt challenging. It might have also brought back memories of when I was first diagnosed. However, I knew it may provide answers and I believed it would completely take me off of my infusion shot so that my body would strengthen and go back to its proper functioning state. I took authority over the fear and stood in God's strength and comfort instead.

On top of this, M.D. Anderson kept telling us that, "As far as we can tell you are cancer free." But Aaron kept asking, "How can you say that if you are not running baselines and retesting so that nothing new has shown up?" So it was also relieving to know that we would possibly get confirmation that all was well.

I knew that there was a reason for this trip. I would meet everyone with a smile and do my best to be a beacon of light to everyone I crossed paths with and let them know how God provided this trip.

Plus, I saw the extra blessings in this trip. I had never been to Chicago, so I was excited! It was an opportunity for me to work my business and meet new people. So I had my notebook and pen in hand waiting to meet new friends! The more my business grew, the more people I would be able to reach with what God has done and is doing in my life, and to be able to glorify Him in all of it.

Many of us are always rushing because we want things done right now, and we think we know what is best. I'm so guilty of that! Well, I don't believe we do know what's best for ourselves most of the time. God's plans and ways are always better than ours, and what we could even imagine. God's plans for us are good and if we could just be people who would put our whole trust in Him and let

Him do His work, could you imagine how many more hearts and lives we could touch?

Yes, we all love the instant gratification of *now*. What if the next time we wanted something we just stepped back, prayed for *His will* to be done, and then left our burden or our want at the cross as His word says? When we give over all control to God, and we put Him in control, that is when true miracles happen and God can be glorified.

I pray if you are reading this that whatever burden you are carrying is put down and given to God right now, and you let Him take control over it – it is not yours to carry, as His word says, my yoke is easy and my burden is light. So give it to Him and let God direct your paths and bless you beyond what you could imagine. That's what I'm doing, and it feels good to let down a burden that is not mine to bear. Find strength in your storm by leaning wholly and fully on God, and you can praise Him through it.

Chapter 28
Cancer Treatment Centers of America

On January 28, 2016 Aaron and I flew to Chicago to Cancer Treatment Centers of America (CTCA) for a second opinion regarding my breast cancer and post-op treatment. My sister Julie was able meet us there from Thunder Bay, even though she could only stay three days. What an experience for all of us. God's hand was over each step, each appointment, each nurse and doctor I spoke with, and every person I came in contact with. What a blessing.

My sister Julie was in awe of CTCA. Since she lives in Canada, seeing how we were treated was a fantastic experience. In Canada the treatment is a bit different. When you need to see a specialist of any sort, there is usually a very long wait, sometimes up to a year. There are many people who will drive to the USA to see a doctor when they feel it's an emergency because they know the wait could be a long time in Canada. That's certainly not the case where I was.

We all got into the Chicago airport and they had a shuttle waiting for us with a driver that gave us all the info we needed as first timers, and I loved it!

We learned quickly how different things were there. When we got to the hotels, as the driver did drop offs, he talked to everyone by name, said something personal to them, and then we went on to the next hotel. There are several hotels that the CTCA puts patients up in, which was amazing!

When it was our hotel, Aaron tried to tip him and he was told that they do not accept any tips there. We were told they are paid very well to take care of the patients and no extra was needed or accepted. That blew my mind, as I had never before heard anyone not take money.

We took our shuttle to the hospital the next day and we were welcomed, and then had breakfast. After breakfast we met with a doctor who had all my files and went over *everything* – it was almost exhausting. However, I knew that the more information they had, the better options they could give me.

They had me in for my MRI, bone scan, blood work; everything I needed, that same afternoon. *Crazy!!!* My sister sat in awe watching how quick everything happened, how kind they were to every single patient, and also how kind they were to the caregivers. As I wrote before, so many people forget about the caregivers, and yet they have such a powerful and important job – the patient's well being.

They found a nodule in my neck and immediately they made the appointment for ultrasound, which lead to a biopsy, all done in the same day. All came back benign. Thank you, Lord.

When we sat with the oncologist, they gave me several options. Several options. At M.D. Anderson, they told me I had *no* other options other than to do the monthly Zoladex shot. Perhaps that was because I was part of a "clinical study." I don't know. Aaron and I discussed that the reason they said I had no options was possibly because I opted to be part of a study to help other patients, and that M.D. Anderson did not want to remove my ovaries since they were worth five years of valuable data.

I was happy to be a part of a study to gather data. However, once my body started suffering they had a professional, ethical, and moral obligation to explore and consider other options. Especially being the world leaders in medicine as they proclaim to be.

One option given at CTCA was oophorectomy. (I had no idea what it was at first – I thought it was an overectomy!!) As she said it, I vividly remembered a dream I had the previous year – a dream I had two or three times and I had even told Aaron about it.

My dream was that something was supposed to come out, and it was clear it was a "woman part." I just never knew if it was a hysterectomy or not. After having that dream, Aaron and I had asked our oncologist at the time if a hysterectomy or an oophorectomy was an option. We were told it was not an option for me because I was pre-menopausal; I did not need it, and it would require more hormone therapy. More hormones? No thank you! So I let it go. There's a reason they say to follow your gut instinct – and why it's important to get a second opinion.

Right away I knew this was the path for me. I felt a complete and perfect peace that I know only comes from God. For whatever reason, I had to go through the past year of this horrible shot and what it did to my body, and I also know everything happens for a reason – it brought me closer to God. It made me lean on God for comfort, strength, and wisdom. I prayed that when God's timing was right that He would open the perfect door that He wanted me to walk through and He did. He opened the door to CTCA and those amazing people.

What blew my mind even more is that when they sent me to see the surgeon, he would not even consider the surgery until I had an ultrasound and MRI to be sure my uterus was in good condition and that there was no sign of anything suspicious.

How thankful I was that they didn't just go ahead with what I decided, but that they were so detailed in each step. They had my well being in mind and wanted to make sure each part of me was checked before I went a step further.

After a few days, Julie went back home and after a week, Aaron and I left to go back to Texas. They said once the results were in that they would book the appropriate surgery for me. I agreed. I left feeling fulfilled. I felt like I was heard and that I was cared for and that I wasn't just a medical record number, but that I was a person, Michelle Perzan.

During that time, I was once again blown away by my friends in the neighborhood stepping up and offering help with all three of the boys. My friend Johanna had them most of the time, since her oldest Matthew and my oldest Daniel were and still are best friends. She had three of her own, so it was like the Brady Bunch for a week!

Just goes back again to how when you let people help you and you are ready to receive it, you will be blessed beyond measure.

Leaving CTCA I felt respected and I had options, exactly what I had prayed for. I was so happy that I waited on God's timing and I didn't push for things that may not have been where I was supposed to be. When the time is right, God always provides, because He is always faithful.

My heart was so thankful that my sister got to come and see the hospital and meet the doctors and see where her baby sister was going for treatment. I'm blessed to have a husband like Aaron who wouldn't take the side effects and the treatment of M.D. Anderson anymore; who reached out and was persistent enough to find CTCA.

When you are in a storm, be grateful every moment for those around you. Be intentional every day, and tell them that you love them and that you're thankful for who they are and all they do for you.

Chapter 29
One Last Surgery

Tuesday, February 23rd, 2016, my friend Stephanie and I flew up to Chicago to CTCA. Since all of my results came back clear and I was told I was cancer free, it was time to be proactive. I was not ever having those shots again and I was happy beyond belief!!!

For this trip, Aaron and I thought it would be easier on the boys if he stayed home, as they were struggling with both of us gone last time and the change in routine was affecting them. They had been through so much the past two years. I know kids are resilient, but I wanted to make life easier for them.

On top of that, when we got back from the first trip to Chicago, Aaron got a staph infection in his face and the doctors told him he should not fly. I believed it was from the stress of watching me suffer. Aaron not being able to come was God confirming that he should stay home with the boys. My sister was not able to meet me there, plus, I needed someone to fly home with since I would be sore, and I wouldn't be able to lift and would need help after surgery while being on drugs.

Two of my friends volunteered, which blew my mind! So my friend Stephanie came with me. Her whole family supported her and me, stepping up to help with her two beautiful girls Madison and Mackenzie while she would be gone helping me. God always provides!

We were picked up in a limo from the airport and it paved the way for the visit. Stephanie could not believe the treatment we received as patients. We drove to Zion with other patients and it was so wonderful to hear their stories and how when other hospitals told them they had no other options, they traveled here and were not only given options, but hope! You could see God working in their lives and it was just so amazing to hear. I loved sharing this experience with a friend.

Pre-op went easy and I even went for a haircut, as they have every need you could want at the hospital – no kidding, there were massages, haircuts, mani's or pedi's – it's spectacular!

As usual, I didn't ask many questions to the doctors, but beforehand I asked Stephanie to go ahead and ask whatever came to mind, because that was usually Aaron's job and I always forgot to ask things! She was prepared, and asked some great stuff that would aid in my short and long-term recovery! She filled Aaron's shoes well.

The next morning we went in and I felt very peaceful; I could feel the prayers from everyone. I was content and thankful I had such a good friend with me that took time out of her life to be there for me. Friends like that are very rare – friends who support you and don't want or expect anything in return. What a blessing. God always puts people in your life at the right time for His glory and it never ceases to amaze me.

The rest is honestly a blur. Apparently the surgery went very well and I was up and walking to the bathroom by myself within two hours of the operation – mostly because I knew from so many C-sections that the quicker I got up, the quicker they would let me go home!

I had to spend the night in the hospital, and my room was like a suite, it was so huge! No joke – you walked in and they had the usual hospital bed, then the television was in an entertainment unit, but then, past that was a couch and a huge area where you could get down and boogie if you wanted to! It was seriously the size of 3-4 usual hospital rooms, and it was quite amazing!

All I did was rest and ate a lot of cherry Jell-O, and that's really all I remember! I did so well that they let me fly home the next day, on Friday.

Aaron was concerned, and wanted me to stay one more day, but they were discharging me anyway. The doctors said I could fly and I wanted to be home and recover in comfort, not in a hotel room. So, the flights were booked and off we went Friday afternoon to the airport, drugged up and ready to roll!

They had a wheelchair for me, and royal treatment once again. All I could think was, all but for the grace of God am I here, being so well cared for. It was God's strength that made me get up and keep pushing myself, to get through the airport terminal and the flight.

My heart knew and I believed that God provided CTCA for me to go to, so what was there for me to worry about? Nothing. He had it all taken care of and I just walked in that faith and victory.

The best part was that I was told I was actually cancer free – it was no longer a guessing game, but a clinical confirmed fact backed up by loads of tests and data. I just wanted to go home.

For me these past few years, there's no other way to get through what I have without complete faith. The times I wander off that, and look at the past years and what has happened, I break down crying, almost in disbelief over everything that has happened and everything I have lost and been through. Some days and weeks were still a struggle for me; especially after a surgery, I found myself far more emotional.

Following this surgery, I was more emotional because I found out afterward that my cousin Tony in Canada had surgery for cancer that had been diagnosed at the end of January. They didn't tell me before the surgery because they didn't want me to worry.

My heart understands why they didn't tell me, but I wouldn't have worried, I would have prayed. However, I totally get why they waited to tell me. It took a couple of weeks to sink in that someone else in my family had cancer, and it brought back a flood of memories of loss and the past few years, and I broke down again. It was a small crack for the enemy to creep in and look at the past in such sadness and loss instead of the amazing healing and blessings that God had provided.

At church the following Sunday I broke down in tears at the end and went up for prayer with Aaron, being open and vulnerable about the past week and how the enemy was trying to creep in and create doubt and fear and loneliness. Saying it out loud took the power away from the enemy.

There will be days that I will continue to stumble, for I am human and I make mistakes every day. I know there will be times that the enemy will continue to try and creep in and remind me of how I suffered, of what I lost, and sadness will follow.

I still don't sleep through the night due to discomfort (because life is never the same after a bi-lateral mastectomy). But I stand strong in prayer because that is when the enemy tries to sneak in and put lies in my head.

I will remember to start each day with prayer and thanksgiving and be grateful for each day God has given me with my boys and with Aaron. I will continue to share my story with others, sharing hope, and God's faithfulness. Life is good and I will persevere.

I pray that God continues to open doors for me to be able to share my story about what God has done for me so that I can encourage others to find strength in their storm just as I did.

Chapter 30
Why Did You Get Cancer, Mom?

One night, I was lying in my bed; it was about a week out of my last surgery, which was February 25, 2016, and my oldest son Daniel was laying with me. We were snuggling the best we could without him touching my tummy, which was still very tender from surgery, so we were holding hands and talking. He asked me, "Mama why did you get cancer? Why do you have to be sick?" Before I could even speak he followed it up with, "You're such a good mama, I don't understand...."

It's not too often at that age they are praising you as a mama, so for a moment I smiled, as these are rare moments that I cherish! I told him that I was happy I went through breast cancer. I assured him again that I am no longer sick; that I have been healed and that God has kept His strong and healing hand over me. I didn't want to go on talking until I felt he understood that he had nothing to worry about or fear.

I shared with Daniel that if we didn't go through trials, tribulations, and hard things, then how do we know what it's like when there's an abundance of good? I told him that we are not able to praise God and reveal what God has done for us if we don't go through challenges and hard times. I explained that because of all the doors God has opened and all of the wonderful doctors and people God has placed in my life, I have been able tell others how my faith has gotten me through my storm.

It was my turn to start asking him questions. I asked, "Hasn't God provided people and amazing hospitals to help Mama? Hasn't God placed an amazing church in our life to pray for us and love us? Hasn't God made sure that I am healed and well and home with you? Hasn't God provided Daddy work from home so that he can help do the things that Mama can't?"

As he answered *yes* to each question, I turned it back around and reminded him that it's so important to be thankful for each thing we go through in our lives because it's what helps us to grow as people, and as children of God. It strengthens us as we learn to lean on God and grow closer to Him. How else do you grow closer to God if you don't have a reason to?

Life's challenges are a way for us to choose our path and what we will do, and whom we will trust in – this world or God.

These are not just words I write; this is how I have had to live my life each day to get through them. I see so much differently than I did two years ago, because of what I went through. I let lots of "little things" go because in the light of eternity they really do not matter.

We do not know how long we have on this earth. We are to make the most of each day and be kind and loving to one another. We are to love our children, enjoy the moments with them, and not say "later...."

We need to live in the *now* and embrace all that God has blessed us with. I say all of this because there are days that are still a struggle for me. I get through them because I know it could be so much worse.

My life will never be the same and I'm not sure I would ever want it to be. Would I love to sleep through the night and wake up refreshed? Yes! Would I love to sleep on my tummy one more time and be able to roll over without waking up, and be able to look at myself and not see scars everywhere? Yes, I would.

They are small things, but things that we take for granted, and once you don't have them anymore, you miss them. However, I am cancer free, and I am blessed with my husband Aaron and three healthy wonderful boys. I have persevered through all of it because of my faith and trust in God, not of anything of this world or anything I have done on my own.

Those scars on my body will always remind me of what a great, loving, healing, faithful Father I have and when I may veer off His lit up path, those scars will remind me to get back on and not take anything for granted. The Lord gives and the Lord takes away, He is all-powerful and I want to always remember that. I have, because *He allows* it.

My son had a fair question – Why? Why my mama? I have made a point to not focus on why. I just thank God that He chose me to be his child, that He has kept His promises of love, comfort, faithfulness, and protection over me and my family. I would not change a thing, as I have grown closer to God in the past two years because of my storm. That is what I focus on.

I smile because He lives in me, and, as the words to the song say, because of Him "I can face tomorrow. I can face uncertain days because Christ lives." I am so thankful for that.

We are called to minister to each other, testify about how God has changed our lives, and show others how trusting in our Lord and Savior Jesus Christ will be sufficient, for his grace is abundant.

Strength in My Storm

Chapter 31
I'm an Ambitious Woman

Looking back, I am so thankful for taking the leap of faith back in 2013 and joining the AWSC with Amy Applebaum and Esther Spina. They have taught me how to be an ambitious woman and how to do it with integrity and success.

Because of the coaching and AWSC, I have grown personally to where I want to speak in front of people and share my story, which is something I had zero interest in before.

In March 2016 Esther asked me to share a speech I did for Toastmasters for an International Contest at the AWC women's conference, which was scheduled for the weekend of April 1, 2016. My speech was about how your faith, positive attitude, and perseverance will get you through whatever "storm" you are going through.

Considering what I shared with you already on my speaking abilities before Toastmasters you may think, "What was Esther thinking – crazy woman!"

Esther has watched me grow and has given me a platform to share my story with others since my diagnosis, and for that I am so thankful.

That weekend came and I was packed, excited, nervous, and thankful for the opportunity. I stepped up to volunteer for the conference, so when I arrived Friday morning, April 1st, I checked into my room, changed into what I would wear onstage that night, and went to help check the ladies in at registration.

At one point, a lady named Kate Rittase came up to me and gave me a hug. She looked familiar, but I didn't remember her name, I guessed I had met her the year before. She told me that she had been watching me for a little bit and hardly recognized me. I looked the same as far back as I can remember, so I asked her what she meant.

Kate told me that I was not the same Michelle she met last year. She told me that I had a confidence about me that she didn't even recognize, by the way I held myself, the way I was walking, and how I spoke. I almost started crying receiving the compliment.

Listening to her and looking in her eyes, she was speaking from the heart. I told her it was strength from God, that He had helped me through so much. I shared with her that I would be speaking a bit later and sharing more, and she told me she could not wait, and knew that I would touch many hearts.

WOW. I was humbled that a stranger, someone I really hardly knew, would say all of that to me.

The conference started, and when my turn came, Esther called my name to come on stage. My heart was pounding out of my chest. I had just come back from the bathroom where I said a prayer and asked for strength and confidence and for God to guide my words and touch hearts.

After taking a couple of deep breaths, I reminded myself that this was about sharing my story to help others. I put a smile on my face and I stood there and spoke with a confidence I never had before, sharing some of me.

Many ladies came up to me to share their stories and talk with me and pray – I loved that part! This year what happened was that other speakers that were there came to me and told me that I touched their hearts and that I did an amazing job. Coming from people that speak for a living really made me smile.

One of the speakers that weekend was Kate… and I had no idea. That was God putting her in my path to instill even more confidence, because when I am up on that stage, it's not about me, it's about sharing my story and what God has done, and showing others that faith is powerful.

This is the weekend that for me it all came full circle – that the decision back in 2013 to hire a coach and learn how to be obedient and let others give to me was showing its value.

Because of the AWC I attend each year, I was able to meet Cassandra Washington in 2015 and become a collaborating author in a bestselling book on Amazon called *Emerge: Real Stories of Courage and Truth* that launched in September 2015.

I would not have had the courage to do that without the coaching and guidance I have gained over the past couple of years and from attending that conference and bonding with other women who truly want to see me succeed.

When I started my Ambit Energy business in 2010 to make extra residual income part time, I had no idea that this would be the vehicle to amazing personal development. It has propelled me to blossom into a vessel for God through my walk with breast cancer.

We had been praying for an opportunity and when it was presented, my ears were open to hear and my eyes were open to see it. You never know how blessings will come, and in my case, it was through this business, as it has opened so many doors for me.

Without the foundation of Christ, I would not be as strong as I am, I would not have the boldness or courage to speak and write and share my story, I would not have been an author or written a blog or a best-selling book, and now to put all of that into this book to share with even more people. I could not have done that without belief in myself, and having complete trust and faith in God as I walked through the doors He opened for me.

I remember now that I am an ambitious woman who is successful as a mother, a wife, sister, aunt, friend, businesswoman, author, speaker, trainer, and coach. I am an entrepreneur in my heart and I'm so happy I was brave enough to step out. I make mistakes because I am human, and that's okay. I learn and attempt to do it better each time.

For me, what's next is whatever door God opens. I believe I will continue to share my story with others, praying that it not only encourages them, but also leads them closer to Christ to show that you can get through any trial, tribulation, or storm when you lean wholly on the Lord and trust in Him.

My heart wants to continue to write and share more parts of my life and journey, parts that were not even touched on in this book, but someone may need to hear. I'm also looking forward to speaking my truths as opportunities arise.

Currently I am feeling better than I have in over two years and that is all thanks and glory to God. I am no longer on any meds at all, and I have not had daily naps since the end of March 2016, which is a huge change in my life. I have enough energy to get through the day.

Not only do I have enough energy, but I am dancing around, smiling, playing the Wii, laughing, and having fun with my family again. I feel like I am starting to get my life back and this is just the beginning, since the meds are almost completely out of my system.

Granted, for a while I was not sleeping through the night and there were days that the lack of sleep caught up with me. However, I knew that too would pass and when I trusted in God, He always gave me the strength to get through each day.

In July 2016 my husband started working with a health and wellness company called Kyani and shared the triangle of health with me. There are only three products: Sunrise, which is juicing in a pouch; Nitro, which helps your body start producing Nitric Oxide again and repairs the body at the cellular level; and Sunset, which is your Omega-3 fatty acids and tocatrienols (aka vitamin e). Since I've been taking these natural supplements, I have only been waking up once per night, and when I do, I go right back to sleep. There have been many nights that I am not waking up at all and that has been such an amazing blessing.

July 10th I travelled up to CTCA in Zion for my three-month check-up and they were going to check my hormone levels, since now that my ovaries were out, there was a high chance of hormone replacement.

All my blood work was done the day before and when I saw the oncologist and naturopath, they told me that all my levels were great. I told them I had been sleeping better. The only thing I had changed was taking the triangle of health from my hubby. They checked the ingredients and confirmed that it was good stuff! Things were looking up!

They said I was good to go and I came back home. The next day, I was volunteering at the Ballard House (which is a place that provides a free place to stay for cancer patients) and I received a text from my hubby telling me he was laid off from work – actually the whole company was being dissolved.

Exactly a week before, I had had another dream, showing me that Aaron would be laid off from his work. I saw who he would be working with and God showed me that it was good – there was so much more I was shown, just so hard to describe. I saw blessings and peace and that it was something that needed to happen and to just trust in Him.

The next morning, I woke up and told Aaron about the dream and said that it would be coming and to just keep trusting in God. Well, exactly seven days later it happened.

Do you know what I saw? I saw that God provided an onshore job for Aaron so we could move to Katy in Dec 2013 – that happened two months before I was diagnosed with breast cancer. Now that I came back from CTCA and I had a clear check-up, the job that God provided was ending, because it was time for a new chapter.

My husband's job was there for the exact time we needed it. He was able to be at every appointment, every surgery, work from home when I was at my lowest points, and cover all my medical needs. That is seeing God's handiwork – and even though it was Aaron losing his income, all I saw was the blessing in it all.

As I write this, he is currently working with a business partner to start a new company. This has been another test of faith and trust, and one that I am just giving completely to God. My eyes and ears were open to see what God showed me July 5th and I'm standing in those promises.

Strength in My Storm

Chapter 32
What Now?

Sharing my story has been a huge part of my healing through my breast cancer. Some people may think it's living it in front of the whole world to see, but for me, after watching how secretive my mom was about her cancer, I knew I had to be different.

I knew I needed support. When someone is secretive, you don't know how to help him or her. You don't know how to pray or what they need. That was so hard for so many others and me with my mom. I wanted to be transparent and really share as much of what I was going through and what I needed as I could, so that if people wanted to help, they could.

Many people have reached out just from my blog posts — some were complete strangers and we are now friends. That is God working. They are people I would never have known if I hadn't stepped out, been bold, and shared my story — as uncomfortable as that was for me.

When things happen to us, we like to hold it in and keep it to ourselves to protect ourselves. There are so many people in the world who go through things feeling alone. If we were to all share, be vulnerable, and speak about how we feel, we would find commonality with so many others. Sharing would help support one another.

Writing and sharing has been a way for me to release how I'm feeling and connect with others who are either going through a similar pain or know someone who is. It doesn't have to be someone with cancer; it can be someone with a burden they are carrying and they are looking for encouragement or a word from the Lord to cling to.

When we share our struggles, others can relate and we can bond together as brothers and sisters in Christ and strengthen and lift each other up. Share your struggle with someone – reach out. So many want to feel like they are not the only one, and something you share may create a bond that may save someone else's life.

God does not want us to hide our challenges from those around us, He wants us to praise Him and glorify Him through our storms. Share your "storm" with someone today. Find support from your spouse, friends, neighbors, or co-workers.

You are not alone, nor should you be, and the more you reach out to others, let them in, and open your heart to receive, the more amazed and empowered you will be at the abundant blessings.

I look back at the past couple years and there were so many days that were challenging; I stand in awe of what has happened and what I have lost. I still cry remembering. Then the clouds always part and God's light shines down and shows me and reminds me of all that He has provided through this "storm," and once again, I smile and Praise Him – I truly do have so much to be thankful for.

For now, I will continue with my passion and work my Ambit Energy and my new HODO business and help Aaron with his Kyani business. I will help with meetings, train team members and whoever is in need, and help others realize their full potential and their dreams. I want to encourage others to find strength in their storm and do my best to guide them toward God by sharing my story. I will watch my three boys, Daniel, David and Dylan grow up, become strong men of faith, have families of their own, and have their own ministries for helping others, and sharing God's faithfulness.

May God's shining light fall strongly on you and may you feel His presence in whatever storm you are going through. May your joy be full and your heart content.

"Life is a storm, my young friend. You will bask in the sunlight one moment, be shattered on the rocks the next. What makes you a man is what you do when that storm comes."

~ Alexandre Dumas, The Count of Monte Cristo

About the Author

Michelle Perzan is an entrepreneur working part of her days in her business in the field of energy, where she helps people save money on their electricity, and the other part with her husband in the health and wellness industry, where they help change lives with nutrition.

Michelle's passion is helping and encouraging others who are struggling in life to see that their faith, perseverance, and attitude are powerful tools. Her goal is to become a speaker for God's glory, sharing her story in the hope of motivating and inspiring others who are experiencing difficulty in his or her life.

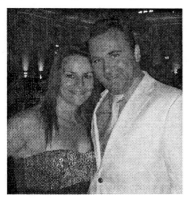

Michelle is happily married to the love of her life, Aaron, and has three wonderful boys, Daniel, David, and Dylan. A Canadian native, she has lived in Texas since 2007, and has made it her home.

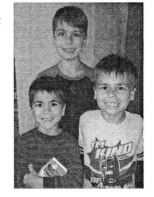

If you are looking for amazing personal development and want to feel more fulfilled, Michelle would love to share with you the business that has changed her life. For more information about Michelle and her work, visit www.michelleperzan.com or email michelle@mperzan.com.